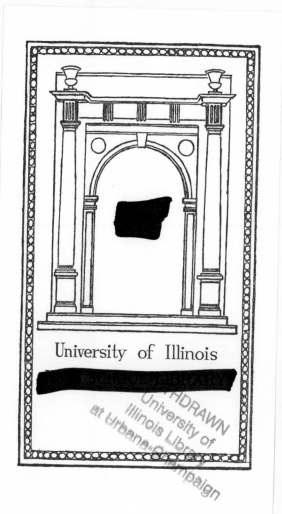

University of Illinois

Creative Insomnia

Creative Insomnia

Douglas Colligan

FRANKLIN WATTS

NEW YORK | LONDON | 1978

Acknowledgments

I am especially grateful to: Dr. Peter Hauri of the Dartmouth Medical School and Drs. Charles Pollok and Arthur Speilman of Montefiore Hospital for their generosity with their time and expertise; to Joyce Fried of UCLA's Brain Research Institute, Anne Harrison of the NTISearch Program, the National Institute on Drug Abuse, and the American Association of Sleep Disorders Centers for their invaluable and speedy help with my research; and to Henriette Gray whose flying fingers were invaluable to finishing the book.

Deserving special mention are: Carolyn Trager, who came up with the idea for this book, and Doug Colligan and the Night Hawks, who proved to me that night people are the best people.

Library of Congress Cataloging in Publication Data

Colligan, Douglas.
   Creative insomnia.

   Includes index.
   1. Insomnia. I. Title.
RC548.C64   616.8'49   78–16578
ISBN 0–531–09901–6

To Louise

Contents

Creative Insomnia

1.
Insomnia as the Enemy and a Possible Tax Deduction

The story goes that one day the nineteenth-century writer and wit Oscar Wilde came home to find one of his least favorite people, the local tax collector, waiting on his doorstep. The man announced he had come to get the property taxes, long overdue, on Wilde's house.

"Taxes?" the writer exploded. "Why should I have to pay any taxes?"

The simple-minded man answered by pointing out the obvious. "But Mr. Wilde, you are the householder, are you not? Isn't this where you live? Where you sleep?"

"Ah yes," Wilde replied, "but you see, I sleep so *badly*."

Creative insomnia at its finest.

In trying for what was probably an historical first—declaring insomnia as a tax deduction—Oscar showed a different, but basically very healthy, attitude toward insomnia that should be an inspiration to us all. Rather than let those sleepless nights degenerate into grim exercises in self-torture, we'd all be better off if we learned to use and, when possible, enjoy the time we suddenly find dropped in our laps.

This is not as far-fetched as it sounds. People are able to cope with insomnia on a level above total misery. Some do it very well, actually leading a kind of double life when sleep deserts them. Others simply learn to use their insomnia as "found" quiet time that they don't get very often. All of them have one thing in common: they know the enemy. That's the first step in dealing with your sleeplessness in any productive way. And it's not as hard as it may seem.

Here's a portrait of a typical run-in with insomnia. You're lying in what used to be your sleeping position, and have been that way for the past hour or so. Your body is tense, a solid knot of muscle. Your mind is spinning at high speed with random, mostly self-defeating thoughts —problems you had today, problems coming up tomorrow, problems you expect *next week*. In the midst of all this your eyelids keep flipping open. The pillow seems too high, too low, too hard, too soft. At some time during the night the sheets turn to sandpaper. Someone has sucked all the air out of the room. You start noticing noises you never heard before.

At this point you flop over into a new, fake relaxed position and lie there suffering a while longer until you drift off to sleep what seems like hours later. Or you may take a sleeping pill that gives you instant sleep and a mind-fogging hangover the next morning. Throughout the next day you are a zombie. You feel as though you never slept. And the worst of it is you start worrying that the next night is going to be a rerun of the night before. You may even lie there convinced that, once again, sleep will make no appearance. This is how many people "cope" with insomnia and end up losing both their sleep and peace of mind.

For years there wasn't really any other choice. Sleep was, in the words of one expert, the "dark continent of the mind," and no one had penetrated very far into its interior. Well, now there's good news. After years of expeditions by a handful of sleep researchers, we've finally got some decent maps. Sleep is not the total mystery it once was, and neither is insomnia. With the discoveries about the causes and treatments of insomnia that have sprung up just in the last ten or fifteen years, there's no reason why you should come out of a showdown with insomnia and be the loser.

What is still one of the big unknowns about sleeplessness is just how many people suffer from it. Educated guesses put the number at about 20 million people, at the very least, and possibly up to 35 million, which is roughly between 10 and 15 percent of the total U.S.

population. Since many insomniacs, unlike Oscar Wilde, prefer to suffer in silence, the real number might be even larger. A 1973 survey of Los Angeles citizens found that a third complained about trouble sleeping and a county-wide poll done in Florida found more than half the people there said they had trouble sleeping. The reason for the difference in the two areas wasn't explained. Maybe the neighbors are a little noisier down South. Whatever the total numbers, you can take some small comfort in the fact that you're not alone in your misery on those nights when you toss and turn.

What *is* known about insomnia is who is likely to get it and what forms it will take. For one thing, it has a slightly sexist bias. Two of every ten women have trouble sleeping as compared with only one of every ten men. Also, people over sixty are more prone to suffer from it, a fact that can be explained, at least partially, by changes in the way they sleep.

When your insomnia does come, it will be in one of three different forms. The first, called *sleep onset insomnia,* is basically trouble getting to sleep. Sleep experts say you can qualify for this kind if it takes you over thirty minutes to doze off at night. Second is *sleep maintenance insomnia,* meaning you can get to sleep, but you can't stay asleep. With this type of insomnia you may find yourself waking periodically during the night. Your wakeups may come hours apart or as frequently as every twenty seconds, depending on their cause. The third, and most devastating, type is *early-morning awakening insomnia.* With this kind you may find yourself alert and miserable at about four or five o'clock in the morning. Most often you can't get back to sleep, and you may succumb to the "dark night of the soul"—hopelessness and depression that sometimes come with this type.

There is a fourth possible kind which is nothing more than a combination of two or, in desperate situations, all three of the insomnias mentioned above. If your insomnia has gotten this complicated, you are probably already looking for professional help to get rid of it. If you're not, you should be.

Even if you have these problems you don't really qualify as a bona fide, serious insomniac unless there is one other feature to your sleep difficulty. It has to interfere with your routine daily functioning. The seriousness of your insomnia is judged not by how long or how little you sleep, but by how well you function the day after. You could spend ten hours sleeping and still feel like a wreck in the morning, or you might spring out of bed refreshed after five hours of sleep.

Too often we let ourselves be brainwashed by all those quaint bits of folk wisdom about sleep, such as, "Get your eight hours every night" and "Early to bed and early to rise makes a person healthy, wealthy, and wise." What makes Ben Franklin such a big expert on sleep? If we all slept the way he recommended, each of us would have to have two beds. He believed a cool bed was conducive to a good night's sleep and for that reason you should always have an extra one ready when your body heated up the first one. Forget Ben Franklin. Only you and your body know the right way for you to sleep and, for that matter, when you genuinely have insomnia.

People have sometimes been talked into thinking they have a sleep problem where none exists. There was one case of a seventy-one-year-old woman who showed up at a sleep clinic claiming she had insomnia or, to be more accurate, that her husband and doctor said she had insomnia. The clinic interviewer asked her why they might think that. "I only sleep three hours a night," she said. How long had this been going on? "Practically all my life," she answered.

She never felt the urge to sleep more, never felt tired, unless of course she had been out all day skiing, which she did often. She never really started worrying about her twenty-one-hour days until her husband and doctor did. She always felt fine but thought that if she was able to get one of those nights of eight hours of sleep she'd heard so much about, she'd feel even better.

After a physical exam, which showed her to be in good shape, she was invited to spend a night hooked up to the clinic's equipment so they could watch her rest. The results showed she had perfectly normal sleep, better than average for someone her age. The diagnosis was that she did not have insomnia but was a "healthy hyposomniac," sleep-talk meaning that she only needed a few hours' rest each night.

Not so long ago the woman would have been labeled an insomniac regardless of how she felt. Doctors flatly assumed everyone had to get seven and a half hours—the average human sleep time—in order to be healthy, wealthy, and wise. No one really knew too much about sleep, except that you had an occasional dream or nightmare and that you'd feel miserable if you didn't get any. There were no ways to examine sleep objectively, no ways to measure what made the difference between good and bad sleep, and no ways to tell why you might have insomnia. No one could even tell you why you needed those seven and a half hours.

A brilliant University of Chicago physiologist changed all this by pioneering sleep research that has uncovered more about the subject in the past twenty-five years than in all the time that came before. The man was Dr. Nathaniel Kleitman, a scientist who spent years of his professional life trying to find out exactly what happens during those hours of unconsciousness that all of us usually take so much for granted.

He was obsessed with the mystery of sleep and poked and probed at it every way he could devise to get the answers he wanted. He and a colleague once spent over a month in the pitch-black depths of the Mammoth Cave in Kentucky to find out what happened when the body was cut off from the twenty-four-hour, sunrise-sunset, day-night cycle. (And he found that the body expanded its "day" to twenty-five hours.) He studied the sleep habits of the Norwegians during the long days of summer and the long nights of winter (and found they slept just like everyone else did, give or take an hour).

His most famous discovery was an accidental one. Technically, it wasn't really made by him, but by a young graduate student, Eugene Aserinsky. In 1956 Kleitman was studying sleep patterns in newborns and gave Aserinsky the job of watching to see if a certain rolling eye motion that infants made at the beginning of sleep was repeated at all during the night. Aserinsky never saw the eyeball roll repeated, but he noticed something else peculiar. Brain-wave records of the infants seemed to show they had awakened, but when he checked on them they were not only still asleep but their eyes were moving back and forth as though watching an invisible tennis match.

When he told Kleitman about this, they started checking other sleepers and found that at some time during the night everyone started watching the same tennis match. This period of rapid eye movement, or REM, sleep came like clockwork four to six times every night. It has a distinct look to it on the brain-wave machine. Recordings seemed to show that the brain was wide awake and working hard. The body was dead still, but the eyes were twitching frantically. Other scientists decided to find out why the brain was working at all.

They began waking up sleepers every time this eye twitching started. Eight out of ten times what they got was a long, detailed, vivid description of a dream the person was having. That's when it became clear that REM time was dream time.

Since then hundreds of sleepers have slept thousands of hours for sleepless scientists who have now managed to piece together a picture of what happens during that big blank spot in your day. It turns out that sleep is a very busy time for both the brain and body. You don't fall into a dead, listless stupor for seven hours or so and then wake up. Your whole system is in an orderly state of commotion during sleep and at any given time is either moving down away from or up toward wakefulness.

Sleep clinicians use different ways to measure this orderly commotion, but the one that seems to give the most exact results is the electroencephalogram, or EEG, which monitors the brain waves and produces a visual record of them. A skilled eye can read a night's record of an EEG and tell what was happening to the sleeper. Even before you are sleeping, when you lie down in bed your brain is already shifting gear. If you are relaxed enough, your brain will be producing alpha waves which, on a print-out, look like a series of tight, even *m*'s. At this point, your mind should start disconnecting itself from the day and set itself loose, free-associating in pleasant fantasies.

Sleep should follow soon, usually within about fifteen minutes. Experts now know that on a normal night you will experience two kinds of sleep, REM and non-REM, which comes first. Non-REM has four stages, or levels. Each is a step deeper into an unconscious state. Your sleep starts with stage 1 of non-REM, the beginning of which is sometimes signalled by a brief twitch in your legs or body, the sign of one last spark of restlessness from the brain. Your stay in stage 1 is very brief, no longer than six or seven minutes, and then you are down to stage 2, which many feel is the true beginning of sleep. At this point your body is more relaxed, your temperature is beginning to drop slightly, and pulse and breathing start to slow. Your brain waves are looser, more relaxed looking than they were in the alpha state and your mind is retreating into itself more. You may have brief flashes of minidreams, disconnected thoughts, and bits of mental flotsam—things to do tomorrow, fragments of a TV show, flashes of the day's events—float through your mind.

Stages 1 and 2 are very shallow parts of sleep. You are easy to wake at this time and if you do get up you'll remember it the next day. This is not true of the deeper levels of sleep, stages 3 and 4, that follow. Sometimes lumped together and called delta sleep after the name of a distinctive brain wave, stages 3 and 4 are the deepest and, some believe, the most refreshing, restorative parts of your night's sleep. They start about a half-hour after sleep has begun and last from a few minutes to as much as an hour.

Stage 4 is as far from consciousness as you'll get in an ordinary day. Your body has slowed way down. Pulse, blood pressure, and temperature have all dropped. Your brain is extremely relaxed and, while you may have a rare dream or two at this time, it will be brief and colorless, usually not worth remembering. It is tremendously difficult to wake you at this time, and if someone manages it, you probably won't remember anything you said or did.

This delta sleep is the time of bizarre behavior, when sleeptalkers sit up and start holding long conversations with themselves and when sleepwalkers get out of bed and begin wandering around. This is also the time of night when children have trouble with bedwetting or with a strange problem called night terrors. Some children have attacks of hysteria and fear and will wake screaming with horror. Very often they won't even remember what caused the panic and by morning none of them even remember waking up. As disturbing as it may be to those that are awakened by these things, the night terror doesn't seem to affect the child in any way. No one knows why these things happen, but the experts say children eventually outgrow the problem.

Once your delta sleep is over, your brain starts to tighten up its wave tempo and head back up toward the more shallow levels of sleep. You have now been out for about ninety minutes and are getting ready to shift into the other kind of sleep, REM sleep. This is as different from being awake as it is from non-REM sleep. It's a state of body and mind so different that some refer to it as a third state of existence.

As REM sleep begins, your body is totally limp. If someone dragged you out of bed and tried to stand you up, you'd collapse like a wet towel. Your body isn't moving at all except for the side-to-side eye twitching discovered by Kleitman and Aserinsky. If you're a man, you start to have an automatic erection; if you're a woman, your vaginal tissue will begin to swell with blood. Inside the body, heart-beat and blood pressure both have jumped, breathing is ragged and irregular, and powerful hormones are pulsing into your bloodstream from places such as your adrenal glands.

At the same time, your brain is electric with activity. In fact, it's difficult to tell the difference between a recording of a fully awake and alert brain and one in REM sleep. All kinds of fantastic scenes and images soar through your mind. This is when you will have most of your dreams and nightmares.

When this REM period is over, so is the first whole sleep cycle of the evening. Then brain and body shuttle over to non-REM sleep and start a new non-REM/REM cycle. In an average night's sleep, a normal healthy adult, age twenty-five to forty-five, has between four and six of these cycles in a steady, predictable sequence. Each half of the night has its own character. The first half has more deep delta sleep, while the second half has more REM (it takes up about a fourth of the night); but the same non-REM/REM shuttle remains constant throughout.

One thing you should realize is that your sleep changes with age. You don't sleep the same way now as you did as an infant, or as you will sleep ten or twenty years from now. We now know that one of the facts of life is that sleep changes with age. Newborn babies spend between sixteen and twenty hours of their days sleeping in four- and five-hour spurts, and spend at least half their sleep in REM dream sleep. Premature infants use even more sleep time, as much as 85 percent, for dreaming, and some believe the sleeping fetus spends all of its time in dreams.

The total hours of sleep time gradually shrink until age twelve, when they settle at around the eight-hour mark. Then, in adolescence, total time starts dropping again and levels off at around seven hours once you hit your mid-twenties. It stays there until you reach your mid-forties, when it starts to diminish once again. By the time you reach your early sixties, you may be routinely sleeping five or six hours a night and doing quite well. Another side effect of getting older is that you have a shallower sleep, with more of stages 1 and 2 and very little of the deeper, delta-wave levels. Sleep is more uneven and we have more awakenings in our sleep after age sixty. It's almost as though we're ultimately programed for insomnia.

Usually these transitions are so gradual that you barely notice them; but there have been a few instances where they have been eerily sudden. Probably the best-documented was the case described by Dr. William Dement, head of the Stanford University Sleep Clinic, in his book, *Some Must Watch While Some Must Sleep*. There was a retired teacher named Professor B. Q. Morgan who lived near Stanford. At one time he had headed the university's Department of Germanic Languages. Morgan told Dement that until the age of twenty-three he had been an average sleeper, getting between six and eight hours of rest each night. At that time he was a graduate student working on his language studies in Germany and had a nightly ritual of going to bed around ten o'clock in the evening.

One night he went to bed at his usual time and, just four hours later, at 2:00 A.M., he found himself wide awake. Since he felt too alert to sleep, he got out of bed and did some studying. The following night the same thing happened. After giving sleep a second chance, he again got out of bed and did some work. He soon found out these four-hour spells in bed had become a permanent part of his life. He had mysteriously changed from an eight-hour sleeper to a four-hour sleeper literally overnight. From that point on, his days were twenty hours long.

Dement was interested but skeptical. Professor Morgan was apparently a well-rested person and, if he did get only four hours of sleep, it seemed to suit him fine. But people sometimes misjudge their sleep time or don't count things such as naps that might affect it. For that reason Dement got permission for one of his staff members to observe a few days in Professor Morgan's life. What he found was that the professor was right. Four hours of sleep was all he needed, and he seemed to thrive on it. His health apparently never suffered from this, and he was able to lead an active life well into his eighties.

Probably the only time you'll ever see a twenty-hour day is when it's foisted on you by a miserable night's sleep, and although there may be times when you can blame your insomnia on some of the sleep changes that come with age, it is hardly ever that simple. The reason is that insomnia is not a disease with a single cure, it's a symptom of many causes, each of which has its own antidote. William Dement likes to compare insomnia to a general ailment like a headache or backache, which could be the sign of one of a hundred different causes ranging from the harmless and ordinary to the dangerous and lethal. According to Dr. Dement, in some ways, medicine's understanding of insomnia today is roughly equivalent to the depth of its understanding of the headache or stomachache about a hundred years ago. Before you get too depressed by this observation, don't forget that most of what we know about sleep has been learned in the past twenty-five years, and at the rate researchers are now making progress, that century's worth of ignorance will be disappearing fairly quickly.

From what's been learned so far, any insomnia you have can be caused by a dazzling array of possible causes. They are usually broken down into three very general categories: physical or medical causes; psychological causes; and a vague group called situational and behavioral causes.

Physical problems that have nothing directly to do with sleep can still keep you awake. Some asthmatics and some epileptics have attacks and seizures at night while they are sleeping. There are some people who only have these problems during the night. Victims of Parkinson's disease, people who are undergoing dialysis or artificial kidney treatments, and those suffering from an untreated hyperthyroid condition all have short, disrupted, and not very satisfying sleep because of their problems.

Migraine sufferers may suddenly wake with a blinding headache that can surface during the REM period of sleep. Ulcer victims can have severe stomach pains at night because, as one group of University of Pennsylvania researchers found, their stomachs pump out as much as twenty times the normal amounts of gastric acid during periods of REM sleep.

A bad heart can disrupt sleep. More than a third of all heart attacks happen during sleep, often while the sleepers are in their REM period. The reason is that part of the night brings with it speeded up heart activity, which could trigger sharp angina pains or even an attack in a weak heart.

It's probably harder to think of a medical problem that couldn't cause insomnia than one that could. Sometimes the cause can be simple but elusive. A classic case of this was the woman who hounded doctors for five years in an effort to eliminate aches and pains around her abdominal area that were so bad they were interfering with her sleep. Elaborate tests at two hospitals turned up nothing suspicious. One doctor's talk with the patient uncovered the fact that her marriage was in trouble. It seemed that the real cause of the problem might be in her head, not her body. He recommended she undergo psychotherapy.

That did no good and, despite the insistence of most doctors that her real problem was she was a hypochondriac, she kept hunting for the "cure." At one point she even checked into a sleep clinic, where they found she really did sleep miserably—no more than four hours of shallow, interrupted sleep on a good night—but they couldn't figure out why. Finally she got the magic cure she was after. One doctor found a constricted blood vessel near her stomach, fixed it with a routine operation, and in the process eliminated her aches, her pains, and her insomnia.

Because of the intensified work of sleep studies, other previously unknown problems that appear only in sleep have been uncovered. For example, there are approximately 100,000 people in the United States who breathe normally during the day but whose whole respiratory system breaks down once they go to sleep. These people actually stop breathing between 400 and 500 times a night.

This odd problem is sleep apnea (which literally means *no breath*) and it was discovered in 1965 by a team of French sleep researchers. It's also been intensely studied in this country by Dr. Christian Guilleminault, Associate Director of Stanford University's Sleep Disorders Clinic and Laboratory. He found that the typical sleep apnea victim is a man, usually middle-aged (among one group of victims the average age was fifty-two), and frequently overweight. Once the victim goes to sleep, his breathing stops for fifteen to thirty seconds. The sleeper then wakes, gasping for air, breathes normally again, and goes back to sleep. About a minute and a half later, the same thing happens all over again.

Incredibly, the victim seldom, if ever, remembers waking. In itself this is not so strange, since most people routinely wake ten or fifteen times every night and never recall doing so. But the apnea sufferer may wake hundreds of times and still have no memory of it. He will feel the effect the next day when he gets up exhausted, as though he got little sleep. Many may have trouble staying awake on the job as a result.

With sleep apnea there is more than a night's sleep at stake. The constant shutdown of breathing raises the blood pressure and could trigger a heart attack. Many men who have apnea have heart problems. Although there's no firm proof as yet, sleep experts also suspect that this ailment, or one like it, is responsible for those mysterious crib deaths in apparently healthy infants.

No one has figured out the *why* of apnea, but researchers do know how it occurs. According to Dr. Guilleminault, it can happen in one of two ways. In the type called upper airway apnea, the windpipe collapses, stopping any air from getting into the lungs. The diaphragm is still working but it can't draw air. In the second type, called central apnea, the diaphragm simply stops working. In some complicated cases, both things can happen at once.

The apnea victim can usually be spotted by two very important symptoms. One is loud snoring, often loud enough to keep his bedmate awake or to keep him banished to another room. Don't start jumping to conclusions if you snore, because there is a second symptom, a washed-out, weary feeling every day, a permanent drowsiness that may interfere with your work. Some people may even remember their waking up. Their bedmate certainly will, since it's usually accompanied with a loud snore.

Very often a doctor can diagnose the problem simply by asking the patient to take a nap. The snoring should come shortly after the patient dozes off. The problem with apnea is not getting it treated—as you will see, sleep clinics do have some successful methods for that—the problem is getting it diagnosed in the first place. Since it is a new problem, some doctors are still not aware it exists. When you complain of insomnia, their first reaction may be to prescribe sleeping pills, which will not only do nothing for your insomnia but could also be dangerous, since they may knock you out so totally that you won't wake up to catch your breath. If you feel worn out and sleepy during the day and your wife complains about your snoring—and if it's apnea-caused snoring she probably will complain—mention the snoring to your doctor. It could help him or her diagnose the problem and keep you from getting a bum sleep cure. The Stanford University sleep clinic had one case of a man who had apnea for thirty years. By the time he arrived at the clinic he had already spent thousands of dollars trying pep pills, sedatives, sleeping pills, and psychoanalysis to eliminate his insomnia.

Slightly more common than apnea but equally mysterious is a sleep problem called nocturnal myoclonus, which involves twitching legs. Once a person has fallen asleep, his or her legs will start twitching once or twice every minute or so for part of the night. With each twitch the victim will wake briefly, for about fifteen seconds, and then go back to sleep. A typical night's sleep may have 300 to 400 of these twitches. By morning the person will feel exhausted but won't know why.

Sometimes the bedmate of the myoclonus victim can help because he or she is the target of twitch-induced kicks. The victims themselves have no way of knowing about these movements and there's no way a doctor can diagnose them without having the patient spend a night in a sleep clinic. The only other clue to the existence of this problem is that occasionally myoclonus victims may feel the need to get out of bed at night to walk off a restless or nervous feeling in their legs.

Don't confuse this problem with that twitch that your legs give at the beginning of a night's sleep. That is a normal and natural part of the sleep process. Also remember that some movement is part of every night's sleep. As you rest you may shift positions about every fifteen to twenty minutes.

Out on the fringes of physical causes of insomnia are some real freaks of nature that include such problems as painful nocturnal erection. This is exactly what it sounds like. When a man gets his REM-sleep-induced erection, he may also be unpleasantly surprised by a sharp pain that comes with it. In the reassuring words of one sleep clinician, the attacks "do not indicate any abnormality in his sexual apparatus." There is no known cause or treatment for this terrifying problem, but there is also no known danger from it.

Another odd problem was spotted by a sharp-eyed scientist, Dr. Harvey Moldofsky of the Clarke Institute of Psychiatry in Toronto, Canada. Some patients came to him complaining of fibrositis, a condition like arthritis, with symptoms of aching bones and muscles, but with no physical signs of any ailment. The people woke feeling stiff and achey in the morning and would limber up as the day progressed.

While watching a group of ten fibrositis victims sleeping in his laboratory, Moldofsky noticed something peculiar about the brain-wave recordings in seven of the people. The deepest part of sleep, delta-wave sleep, was polluted with alpha brain waves usually only found in the alert, relaxed brain. Tests with other fibrositis sufferers have turned up similar brain-wave pollution. The two big questions now are: "Why does this happen?" and "How can these brain-wave leaks be plugged up?"

There is one other physical problem you should know about that doesn't cause insomnia but may make you feel as though you're not getting enough sleep. It's called narcolepsy. It's a strictly physical ailment that triggers sleep attacks in its victims. Without warning, a narcoleptic instantly drops into a state of dreamy REM sleep and stays that way for ten or fifteen minutes. In a typical day a narcoleptic can have as many as twenty of these sleep attacks.

Among the symptoms that often accompany narcolepsy is total body paralysis when narcoleptics wake in the morning. For as long as five or ten minutes all they can move are their eyes. Cataplexy, the total collapse of all muscles, is another symptom. These collapses can be triggered by any stress or strong emotion. Narcoleptics have suddenly toppled over while making love, spanking their kids, or even laughing at a good joke. There is one case on record of a narcoleptic fireman who had a cataleptic attack while climbing a ladder to a burning building. One last common symptom is having vivid dreamy hallucinations during the sleep attack. "It was a monster with great red glowing eyes that were blinking at me. It sat there breathing smoke in my face," was how one woman narcoleptic who had a sleep attack while driving in the middle of New York City traffic described the "dream" she had about the taillights and exhaust of the car in front of her.

You can also have some of these symptoms and not have narcolepsy. Nodding off at a dull business meeting or, God forbid, at the wheel of your car does not add up to narcolepsy if it is not a daily problem and these sleep attacks are not uncontrollable. Even something as bizarre as morning paralysis is not necessarily a symptom of narcolepsy. Canadian Eskimos routinely suffer sleep paralysis but not narcolepsy. The reason why they can't move in the morning isn't clear, although one theory is that it may be a psychosomatic by-product of the fact that, as a culture, they repress all emotions. You may occasionally experience paralysis when you wake after a normal night. If this should happen, wait a few minutes and the paralysis will clear. You can speed up the process by first blinking your eyes quickly, and then concentrating on loosening your body muscles, starting with your face and working down.

Where there is genuine narcolepsy there is usually genuine suffering as well. Narcoleptics are often labeled as dull, lazy, or stupid because of their constant sleep attacks. It causes real hardships in their social life and on the job, if they can get one. One young man, a narcoleptic, was taken out to dinner as part of a job interview with a prospective employer. During the meal he suddenly had a sleep attack and fell face first into a plate of spaghetti. Another narcoleptic lost his computer programmer's job because he punched the wrong keys during a sleep attack and caused hundreds of thousands of dollars in equipment damages. And then there was the narcoleptic night watchman who, for obvious reasons, couldn't hold down a job.

There are an estimated quarter of a million people in the United States with this particular sleep problem. Many routinely spend fifteen years looking for help before they finally find it at a sleep clinic. There they get drugs that help fight off sleep attacks, usually stimulants of some kind, and, if they also have cataplexy, special suppressants to take care of that.

Physical problems cause their share of insomnias but they don't make up the biggest group of causes. That honor belongs to insomnias that come from your mind. Doctors, for example, have known for years that serious psychological problems include insomnia among their side effects. The nights of seriously depressed people and of manic-depressives are as miserable as their days. Once the mental illness disappears, however, so does the insomnia.

But the range of psychological problems that can cause insomnia extends far beyond serious mental illness. The evidence that is in now indicates that almost any psychological problem, from the very mild to the very serious, can ruin sleep. In serious cases, this insomnia can take on a very distinct form.

There is one very special type called REM-interruption insomnia that usually plagues someone who managed to survive some emotionally devastating experience but continues to dream about it. Concentration camp survivors often suffer this way, as do others who went through a huge emotional trauma, such as losing most or all of their family in an accident. After a while the dread of reexperiencing these dreams, or, more accurately, nightmares, is so strong that the person automatically wakes up at the beginning of each of his or her REM dream periods.

One sleep researcher characterized it this way: "It is not that common a phenomenon and usually only appears in people who have been deeply traumatized. They have nightmares all their lives. Sometimes they may not even remember the content of their dreams, but they awaken with a sense that something terrible has happened to them. They may or may not have trouble falling back asleep, but they'll wake up over and over again."

Usually the trauma that caused the sleep problem is dug in so deeply that no amount of psychotherapy is capable of working it free. The only method that works with any success, say sleep clinicians, is a steady program of tranquilizers.

If your insomnia does have psychological roots, it's probably from problems that are less devastating. Everyday difficulties claim many more casualties and do much more damage to sleep. You probably already know from your own personal experience that almost any kind of stress, good or bad, can wreck part of a night's rest. Family problems, divorce, the illness or death of someone close, problems at work, not having any work, all have a way of preying on your mind as you lay there in bed waiting for sleep to come. Even happy events—an upcoming vacation, a wedding, the prospect of an exciting new job—can have the same miserable effect.

When the stress disappears, usually the insomnia disappears right along with it. Once you get that job or once your spouse is out of the hospital and recovered, you stop worrying and start sleeping better. Unfortunately, this does not happen all the time. After a while you may forget about what caused the insomnia and instead get caught up in the problem of insomnia itself. At this point a kind of self-perpetuating thought process springs up. You start worrying about losing sleep and then end up losing more sleep because you are worried.

You lose your perspective on how bad your problem really is and become obsessed with your sleeplessness. A group of University of Maryland researchers found this out when they compared one group of insomniacs with a similar group of normal sleepers. Even though the insomniacs only slept an average of forty-three minutes less than the normal sleepers, they were convinced that every night's sleep was almost nonexistent and, considering how mild their problem really was, they were overly preoccupied with sleep. Their attitude could be summed up in the remark made by one cheerless soul: "I never know when I'm going to have a really horrible night's sleep, or just my usual lousy one."

The reason so many insomniacs feel this way, according to Penn State psychiatrist Dr. Anthony Kales, is because they're depressed. In a survey of insomniacs at the university's Sleep Research Treatment Center, which Kales runs, he found that well over four-fifths of the sleepless had noticeable psychological problems, usually depression. They were worried people, discouraged and low in self-esteem. Given this state of mind, it's no wonder they succumbed to the vicious-cycle effect of insomnia.

Sometimes it takes nothing more than being depressed to keep your insomnia going. There are those, like Dr. Kales, who believe a depressed state of mind is the single most common cause of insomnia. Many doctors routinely look for signs of it in their insomniac patients, and some even prescribe antidepressants instead of sleeping pills to give their patients rest. If you feel this is what is at the root of your sleeplessness, your best bet is to head for a doctor's office if the insomnia is more than two weeks old. He should be able to help or refer you to someone who can.

The strangest of all the psychological insomnias is a ghostly group labeled pseudo-insomnias. These are "nonproblems" that defy any explanation. As sleep study techniques have gotten more sophisticated, the number of insomnias included in this group has been shrinking over the years. They turn out to be cases of alpha-wave pollution, subtle medical problems (e.g., the woman with the blocked blood vessel), or, as one University of Chicago research group discovered, cases where people's minds tend to be hyperalert even while they sleep, making them think that they sleep less than they do.

Still, insomnias do turn up that baffle the experts who try to cure them. Stanford University sleep doctors had one problem case like this. It was a sixty-one-year-old physics professor who said he had had trouble getting a decent night's sleep ever since he was at college. Practically every day of his life he spent in a stupor. Because of this, his work suffered badly and he decided to retire from teaching early, at age fifty-eight.

That still left him with his insomnia. To get help he went to the Stanford Sleep Clinic, where they asked him to keep track of how long he slept each night for two weeks so they could see how bad his problem was. Two weeks later he reported his average sleep time: 3 hours and 59 minutes. "It seemed clear," said Stanford's Dr. William Dement, "that Mr. S. had a terrible sleep disturbance."

Mr. S. then spent four nights in the sleep laboratory, where clinicians could monitor his sleep with their machines. The results didn't come close to what the professor had recorded. Each night in the laboratory he slept a peaceful eight hours, a fact he just couldn't believe at first. Neither he nor the sleep experts could offer any explanation why there was an almost four-hour difference between his perception of sleep and the sleep lab's records. Although he still felt as though he had serious insomnia after this, the man no longer worried about his sleep as obsessively as he once did and felt a little less worn out during the day after he got the news about the eight-hour nights.

There was a time when such people would automatically be labeled hypochondriacs, given a few sleeping pills, and sent home. Now sleep experts are saying it's more likely they are suffering from insomnia caused by reasons not yet uncovered. With the level of expertise sleep clinicians now have, this group of "pseudos" is fast becoming an endangered species in the world of insomniacs.

What can be almost as elusive and mysterious are the insomnias with behavioral or situational causes. Some of these are fairly obvious. You already know, for example, that the first night's sleep in a strange place is usually a poor one. People living near airports or heavily traveled roads or streets may not sleep as well as someone living on a quiet country road or in a peaceful part of suburbia. Various studies have uncovered the fact that, while people who share the same bed may have a good sex life, often they'd get a better night's sleep if each dozed in a separate bed, especially if one of them happens to be a restless sleeper. Sharing your bed with someone can mean sharing your insomnia as well. Finally, you may occasionally be a victim of what's known as "Sunday Night Insomnia," usually the result of changing your bedtime schedule on weekends by going to bed later and getting up later.

Carelessness with everyday drugs can also ruin your sleep if you're not aware of how you abuse them. Caffeine is probably the one that's the most taken for granted and, as far as wrecking sleep goes, the most abused. Depending on your sensitivity to the "up" effect of this drug, one cup of coffee can have a stimulating effect on your brain for as long as seven hours after you drink it. Some people routinely drink ten to twenty cups of coffee every day and never see a connection between that drug habit and their insomnias. Others may be keeping themselves awake with slightly weaker doses of caffeine, which is a standard ingredient in beverages such as tea, cocoa, and cola drinks.

If you're a heavy smoker—that is, two packs or more per day—your nicotine habit may also be keeping you up. Researchers have found that some smokers, after they've been asleep about four hours, will go through nicotine withdrawal that is so strong they'll wake up craving a cigarette. If you're a heavy smoker trying to kick the habit, you may also lose a little sleep over it. One U.S. Public Health Service survey of smokers who did manage to quit showed that close to a third of them complained of insomnia as one of the aftereffects. Fortunately, the insomnia in this instance is a temporary one.

Another sleep-damaging drug—one that has 70 million users and generates about $10 billion worth of business each year—is alcohol. As a nightcap, alcohol eventually loses its punch, and you have to keep drinking more and more to get the same effect. In large quantities— after a real binge or in the extreme case of the alcoholic—it can ruin normal sleep for months or years. In any quantity, alcohol wipes out the REM periods in your sleep and delivers a shallow, uneven rest. When you stop drinking, all that suppressed REM sleep will come surging back, bringing with it a glut of dreams or even nightmares bad enough to cause insomnia.

You may also be taking prescription drugs that are solving one problem while causing another—insomnia. Diet pills (or appetite suppressants, as they are officially known) keep your hunger down and your alertness up, sometimes to the point where you can't get to sleep if you take the pill late in the day. Antidepressant drugs such as Dexedrine and Ritalin can have the same effect and, like alcohol, wipe out your REM sleep as well.

Sleeping pills can take an ordinary, everyday little insomnia and turn it into a real monster. The reason is very simple. Sleeping pills can cause the very problem they were designed to cure. Taken nightly, they only work for a short time, usually no longer than two weeks. You will get more grisly details later, in the chapter devoted to the sleeping pill, but for now all you really need to know is that if you take prescription sleeping pills long enough, your insomnia and the quality of what little sleep you do get will both be *worse* than when you were taking no pill at all.

Okay, you say, I don't smoke, don't drink, don't pop pills, sleeping or otherwise, and I still don't sleep well. If this is the case, maybe you're a self-taught insomniac. What sometimes happens to people is that they have trouble sleeping for one reason and, once that reason disappears, retain that insomnia like a bad bedtime habit. Suppose you suddenly get a new job with a high salary, a lot of responsibility, and a lot of headaches that keep you awake and worried at night. After a while, the crown lies a little more easily on your head, you wield your power with a sure hand, and have fired everyone who gave you those headaches. But you can still have your insomnia if every time you step into the bedroom all you see are reminders of those sleepless nights: the clock you'd stare at until three in the morning, the lamp you'd click on for late-night reading, the bedside table where you kept the sleeping pills that didn't work, and, of course, the bed where you lay so long and slept so little. This habit of thinking is called conditioned insomnia and it can be as devastating as the original cause of your sleeplessness.

The surest sign that this is your problem is if you sleep fine in any bedroom but your own. The stranger your surroundings, the better you'll sleep. One young man who had this problem, a twenty-year-old college student, had insomnia since he was a child, the result of years of lying in bed kept awake by the violent, late-night screaming matches his parents had. He found it practically impossible to get a good night's sleep at home and didn't do much better at school.

The best sleep of his life came during a mountain climb he was making with some friends. Sunset came before he was able to reach the summit, and he had no choice but to stop right where he was for the rest of the night. Unfortunately, it was on a narrow stone ledge in the face of a cliff. To keep from falling off the mountain he had to tie himself to the rock before settling down for the night. And there, dangling from the face of a cliff miles away from his home, his cursed bedroom, and the reminders of his screaming parents, he quickly fell into a deep, totally refreshing sleep—the best he had all year.

Another reason you could have insomnia is that you have Zeitgeber problems. Zeitgebers (literally, "timegivers") are subtle and not-so-subtle time cues that help your body clock, which regulates when you sleep and when you wake, follow a consistent, steady schedule. Anything from the cycles of day and night and what time you get up for work, to when you eat your meals can be Zeitgebers. Your body clock is sensitive and needs these reassuring cues to keep in step with the day. When you confuse your body clock, you throw off everything from your appetite to normal sleep habits, with insomnia as the final result.

Jet lag is probably the most common way to throw off your body clock with new Zeitgebers. Your body may be in Paris, but your internal clock will still be in Chicago. That is why for the first few days in a new time zone you will feel like sleeping when everyone else is awake, and why you'll feel like eating when they don't. Usually, after about three days or so, you are resynchronized with local time.

You can experience the same miserable effects of jet lag without flying to Europe. Just change your work shift. This is particularly hard on your body, since you're fighting the two biggest Zeitgebers of all, night and day. According to the United Nations International Labor Organization, about a tenth of the world's work force live this way and suffer the consequences of completely inverting their sleeping and waking habits. The most common complaints of shift workers the world over are that they have indigestion problems when they're awake, and are awakened by hunger pangs when they're asleep. They also sleep less, an average of an hour and a half, every night.

Fortunately, your body clock is highly adaptable, and if you give it enough time to set it from one steady routine to another, the sleep problems will usually disappear after a brief adjustment period. Night workers, for example, can usually attune their bodies to a new schedule within three weeks of the changeover. Where some people make a mistake is in trying to straddle the two shift schedules, as in working nights during the week and living on a day schedule on the weekend, or by totally ignoring the body's need for some kind of a routine.

If you don't give your body some kind of schedule, it's going to get even with you. Dr. Quentin Regestein, head of the Sleep Clinic at Boston's Peter Bent Brigham Hospital, had one patient whose sleep was a casualty of just such carelessness. He was a fifty-three-year-old policeman who claimed he never got a decent night's rest and who barely managed to make it out of bed every day at 8:30 A.M. Morning was always the worst part of his day. His brain never really got started until late in the afternoon. He seldom got more than four or five hours rest every night and occasionally tried to catch up by going on sleep binges, sleeping from nine o'clock in the evening to noon the following day.

A few questions turned up some of the reasons why his sleep was so elusive. For one thing, he routinely drank twenty cups of coffee each day to wake himself up and keep himself going. Secondly, he was so hyperalert from all the caffeine still in his system that he wouldn't try going to bed at an early hour. Bedtime fluctuated between 2:00 and 3:00 A.M., never earlier. His cure was simple and effective. He had to cut back on his coffee and go to bed at a fixed time, 12:30 A.M. Within a few weeks he was sleeping soundly.

Of course there are always circumstances beyond your control that can disrupt your sleep. For example, if you're indecisive about when to turn your air conditioner on some summer nights, you might be interested to know that in rooms hotter than 75 degrees Fahrenheit people sleep less well. Weather can trigger insomnia in some sensitive people who become restless and agitated when the barometer is recording extreme highs and lows. And of course there is the curse that comes with living in thin-walled apartment buildings or near busy airports—noise.

Just how much insomnia can be caused by noise depends on how familiar a sound is, how loud it is, how long it lasts, and how sensitive you are to it. You're more susceptible in the early, shallow stages of non-REM sleep and during the second half of the night, when sleep in general is lighter. And some people are naturally more sensitive to sound because they are such light sleepers. A person's sex can also make a difference—women appear to be more sound-sensitive than men. Age can be a factor, too. The sleep of people over sixty is naturally shallower, a fact that makes them more liable to wake up when exposed to a sound that ten years before might not even have caused them to stir.

Familiarity with and sensitivity to certain noises also make a big difference. This explains why, for example, some parents may sleep through a window-shaking thunderstorm but wake at the slightest whimper from their baby. For some people, a certain quota of racket is necessary to get a normal night's sleep, as city people who move to the country soon discover.

One person's lullaby may be another's insomnia, however. One woman found this out the hard way from her neighbor, the mad barker. Almost every morning, at about 3:00 A.M., her telephone would start ringing. When she stumbled out of bed and answered it, she would hear a man on the other end barking. The calls came often, almost every night, and they were beginning to take their toll on her sleep and her sanity. Finally she complained to the phone company.

After a few tries they managed to trace the calls to a neighbor of hers. He explained that the woman's dog had a bad habit of howling at three in the morning and waking him. Not wanting to suffer alone, the man would call the woman and bark at her every time her dog got him up. When she heard the explanation for the strange calls, the woman muzzled her dog at night and in the process assured everyone an uninterrupted night of peace and quiet.

What are the dangers of insomnia? What does losing one night's sleep do to you? Sleep researchers have kept everyone from the traditional laboratory rat to willing people awake night after night in experiments to find out what happens to the body without sleep. Early experiments with animals made insomnia look like the next ultimate weapon. Dogs deprived of sleep for a little more than a week suddenly died. Cats lost all control over their appetites and would sit in front of food dishes for hours, eating past the point of reason like food-devouring automatons. Rats went totally berserk and turned into vicious, cunning cannibals.

By comparison, people turned out to be a big disappointment. No one died or ate anyone else. No one sat in a restaurant eating for hours. The wide range of responses to losing sleep at first made it difficult to conclude anything about the effects of insomnia. After years of work, the experts now have two major conclusions to make about losing all of one night's sleep. The first is the not-too-startling finding that going one night without any sleep at all was certain, in the words of one report, to "increase the 'unhappy mood' content" of your day. In other words, you would most likely feel miserable the day after a bad night.

The second, more encouraging finding was that even losing all of a night's sleep has practically no effect on how well you function the next day. After elaborate tests in which sleepless volunteers were asked to add tedious columns of numbers, play complicated war games, do monotonous counting exercises of images flashing in front of their eyes on TV screens, and do elaborate math problems, sleep experts found that even after going four days with no sleep people have been able to do very complicated mental jobs accurately and efficiently if left to work at their own pace. Only when asked to do boring, monotonous jobs did the sleepless show signs of slipping.

More sophisticated techniques of sleep monitoring now indicate that the body doesn't allow itself to lose sleep beyond a certain point. People who have been sleep-starved continually have quick, flickering spells of what are called micro-sleeps, automatic lapses into sleep that last a few seconds. The longer a person is forced to go without sleep, the more of these micro-sleeps he or she is likely to have. It's as though the body has its own compensating device.

From the scientific evidence gathered so far, it looks like most people overrate the damage of losing one night's sleep, and underrate the resilience of their bodies to adjust, given half a chance. If you relax and let it surface, sleep will come on its own, no matter where you are—dangling off the face of a cliff, in your own bedroom at home, or even free-floating in the alien world of space. During their months in space, Skylab astronauts slept as well in the eerie zero gravity of their space habitat as they did in their bedrooms on earth.

On most nights, you should be able to sleep the sleep of the astronauts. When you can't, you can take some comfort in the fact that whatever is causing your insomnia is likely to be a relatively minor problem that will disappear in a few days. Don't make your insomnia worse than it is by brooding over it. Many short-term insomnias have been promoted to long-lasting ones this way. Usually your body and brain can recover quite nicely without your having to worry about it. The evidence now is that the most you stand to lose after a bad night's sleep is some of your daily quota of natural ebullience.

When it comes to dealing with insomnia, a little knowledge is not a dangerous thing, but a lot is even better. Having some understanding of the causes and effects of sleeplessness is only part of the battle. You should also know how your personal sleep system operates, how much rest you need, and when you need it. And that is where the next chapter can help.

2.

You and Your Sleep Hunger: How Much Sleep Do You Need?

She's identified only as Miss M., a seventy-year-old retired nurse who liked to work at her hobbies of writing and painting to fill her spare time. And Miss M. had a lot of spare time—about twenty-three hours a day. Ever since she was a child she found she could do quite well on about an hour's sleep a night. If she were really exhausted, she sometimes slept a little longer, maybe an hour and a half or so.

British sleep researcher Dr. Raymond Meddis met Miss M. through an ad he had placed in local newspapers saying he was looking for people who were able to function on very little sleep. To find out if Miss M. was accurate about her sleep, he asked her to do two things. The first was to keep careful track of her sleep time, including naps, if any, for two weeks, using a sleep diary. The second was to come to his sleep laboratory for eight nights so he could watch her sleep.

Her diary showed she averaged about fifty minutes sleep a day without the help of any naps. In the sleep lab, the results were about the same. The first two nights she didn't sleep at all, but she made up for lost rest by sleeping extra time the third night, a total of ninety-nine minutes, mostly in the deep stage-3 and stage-4 levels of non-REM sleep. After that, she averaged just a little over an hour's rest every night. A restless, energetic woman, she told Meddis she despised inactivity and simply couldn't understand why other people could waste so much valuable time in bed.

And then there is Mrs. O., a fifty-two-year-old nurse who can't get along on less than twelve hours' sleep and often logs sixteen hours in bed. It's a problem she's had since high school, where she learned to go out only on dates where there would be a lot of activity to keep her awake. If she went to the movies she'd fall asleep halfway through the picture. When caring for her children as babies, she'd only feed them while lying on the floor, to eliminate the danger of dozing off and accidentally dropping them. She could play with them but could not do quiet things, such as help them with their homework. If she tried, she'd nod off. The only way she could stay awake on the job was to work in the busiest, most hectic part of the hospital.

She too ended up in a sleep lab. The first night she put in what was for her a short night's sleep of eleven hours. Another night of only nine hours sleep left her totally exhausted the next day. An elaborate checkup showed that she was perfectly healthy and had no sleep disorder. Her only problem was that she needed at least twelve hours sleep to get by. Sleep doctors at Dartmouth Medical School's sleep clinic helped her enjoy more of her day by cutting back her sleep with a special-dosage program of amphetamines. With this program she was able to sleep a fairly normal eight hours and, incredibly, never developed an addiction to the drugs, even two years later when examined again.

It's probably safe to say that somewhere between Miss M. and Mrs. O. is your ideal sleep time. All you've got to do is find it. If you get the average American's night's sleep, you already have your answer—seven and a half hours. Since statistical averages don't tend to exist in real life, your personal sleep time probably hovers somewhere above or below this number.

For most sleepers the time is less than the seven-and-a-half-hour average, according to University of Florida sleep expert Dr. Wilse Webb. He's found that the majority of people sleep less than seven hours, and in one survey he discovered that many of us are sleeping about an hour and a half less than our grandparents did sixty years ago. A faster pace of living is getting us all out of bed sooner; television, with its late-night movies and post-midnight talk shows, is getting us to bed later; and the big Zeitgeber in the sky, the sun, has been eclipsed by the electric fixtures that light up our homes and favorite all-night grocery stores. For better or for worse, we've all gained more control over sleep than ever before.

Certain aspects of sleep will always be beyond our control. As mentioned before, age is the single biggest factor in how long we sleep. Our needs gradually go down from the time we're born, leveling off to eight hours by age twelve, to seven hours between our mid-twenties and late forties, and then taking one last dive, until by our sixties and seventies we routinely get by on five and six hours' sleep. Sometimes these changes come almost yearly, especially during that stretch of agony known as the teen-age years. In one survey of nineteen-year-olds, Dartmouth psychologist Peter Hauri found well over a third of the people polled said they routinely got up to two hours less sleep than they did as sixteen-year-olds.

Other temporary physical changes bring their own temporary shifts in your sleep appetite. Pregnant women may sleep as much as two hours longer than usual during the first three months of pregnancy. This bonus tends to disappear in the course of the pregnancy, and the last few weeks could be just the opposite—restless nights with very little sleep.

The way sleep needs change has always fascinated Dr. Ernest Hartmann, a sleep expert from Tufts University and director of the Boston State Hospital Sleep and Dreams Laboratory. After years of study, he's worked up a scorecard of what are the good and bad influences on a night's rest. Most of what he found probably confirms what your common sense or own experience has already taught you.

People whose bodies have gone through some stress or change, such as an operation, an illness, or injury, seem to need more sleep. Not only pregnant women, but many others who are approaching their premenstrual period may also find they need to sleep more. A stretch of unusually hard physical work or even going on a diet can also result in more sleep time.

Emotional and mental stress from adjusting to the pressures and demands of a new job, more brain work required around exam time, or recovering from the aftershock of losing someone through divorce or death—all seem to drive us to seek the comfort of sleep. For example, the most common reason for spending more time in bed, according to one group of women college students that Hartmann surveyed, was boyfriend trouble. In another instance, Hartmann had a college student complain that he just couldn't function on his old sleep quota. He needed an extra one or two hours a night to get through the day. The student was a thirty-year-old man who had worked as a manual laborer most of his life before getting into college as part of a special program for those naturally gifted with high intelligence. Not used to the heavy mental work of college, the man needed more sleep to cope with the added intellectual effort, Hartmann says. In general, any kind of pressure that is going to leave you physically, emotionally, or intellectually drained will probably also leave you hungry for more sleep.

Not surprisingly, the opposite is also true. Being in good physical shape and keeping your weight stable will also keep your sleep appetite down. This explains why people who start exercising regularly by running, for example, often find they not only sleep better than before they started exercising, but they sleep less as well. Being in good psychological shape has the same effect. That is why you may find you are actually sleeping less during an especially relaxing vacation and why, Hartmann says, people who have successfully completed psychotherapy may also find they are spending less time in bed.

These kinds of influences only make temporary shifts in your sleep routine. The effects of a bad week at the office or a great two weeks at the shore fade in time. What lasts, what you have to live with each night of your life, is your sleep personality. You not only have a built-in need for a certain amount of sleep every night, but you have your own style of sleeping as well. Finding out what these are not only will spare you some unnecessary insomnia but will help you harmonize your daily life with your night's rest.

Because there's no simple way to characterize any person's sleep style, sleep experts have had to take it apart and study it one piece at a time. For example, Ernest Hartmann points out that the number of hours you spend in bed can put you into one of two time groupings: the short sleepers (less than six hours per night), and the long ones (eight and one-half hours or more). In studying the two groups, Hartmann found there were definite personalities that went with each.

Typically, short sleepers are dynamos, persons of action who are energetic, ambitious, always on the go, doing twenty things at once. On personality tests they score normal or even above normal in the way they respond and conform to the standards of society. Short sleepers are not usually worriers. They don't have time to brood about their problems. When problems do plague them, they lose themselves in their work. Many successful politicians, businessmen, and career soldiers make up the ranks of the short sleepers. Winston Churchill was a shortie.

On a scale of normalcy, Hartmann says, long sleepers tend to be a "slightly sicker group" and harder to typecast. As a group, they are mildly neurotic, more critical of the standards and demands of society, and more introspective. They seem to be always revising and questioning their ideas and often use sleep as an escape from the problems of the day. In a word, they are worriers. They make excellent artists, writers, and philosophers, but the message here seems to be: Don't follow long sleepers into battle or elect them president. If you're a long sleeper and want to drop a name, try Albert Einstein.

"In computer terminology," Hartmann says, "short sleepers are pre-programmed. They had already established their program for activities. Long sleepers were frequently re-programming themselves. Their re-programming during the day might require more restoration at night." This could explain, he adds, why the long sleepers seem to have more dream sleep, to give their brains more time to mull over and splice the constant flow of new ideas into their thought circuits.

Beyond the long and short of your sleep, there is also the tantalizing question of whether or not your personality is related to how well or poorly you sleep. In 1965 a young sleep researcher named Lawrence Monroe, who was working on his psychology doctorate at the University of Chicago, decided to find out why some people were so much better at getting a good night's rest than others. After an elaborate sifting and sorting process, he got two groups of men of mixed ages and backgrounds to volunteer as guinea pigs for a very special test.

Using one of the sleep researcher's most valuable tools, the newspaper ad, he recruited men who slept well and those who slept poorly but did not complain about insomnia. He gave both groups a battery of physical and psychological tests and then had them sleep in his laboratory while he and his machines watched. As expected, the good sleepers made the most of the seven hours they were allowed to stay in bed. They averaged about six and one-half hours of sleep per night, while the poor sleepers got an average five and three-quarters hours.

The two groups were not only different in the amount of time they slept but in the way they slept as well. Poor sleepers periodically skimmed much closer to the surface of wakefulness during their night's rest. In general, they had a much shallower sleep with more of the first two stages of sleep and fewer of the deeper, delta-sleep stages than the good sleepers. Their bodies seemed much more alert than the bodies of the average sleepers. They had higher temperatures and pulse rates, tossed around more at night, and even woke up more —all signs of a hyperaroused mind and body.

One of the big surprises of the study came from a question put to the members of each group before they went to sleep. Monroe and his fellow sleep-watchers asked: "How long do you think it will take you to get to sleep?" The good sleepers said, "about seven minutes." And they were right. The poor sleepers said, "Oh, probably an hour or so." It took them fifteen minutes.

On the psychological profiles, the poor sleepers came out as being more introverted, more emotionally disturbed, and a little more anxious than the good sleepers. In a word, they were worriers, very much like Ernest Hartmann's long sleepers.

If you find that you fit in this group, it is also possible you may be prone to insomnia as well. The reason is that some of these same characteristics have turned up in many groups of insomniacs. In talking to insomniacs from Los Angeles, for example, psychiatrist Dr. Anthony Kales found they tended to be individuals who were somewhat shy and a little inhibited, the kind of people who tended to hold in their anxieties rather than act them out.

One of the effects of bottling up all these worries is that the insomniac personalities always carry their distractions and pressures inside themselves. The result is often that they are so self-distracted that they are not very aware of what's going on around them. This inner pressure is so strong that doctors have found many insomniacs seem to have erratic reactions to stimulations and seem more sensitive to distractions of noise and light around them. Insomniacs are so overstimulated by their own worries that they deliberately avoid any more stimulations outside themselves. Thus, they may even lead much quieter, less eventful lives than noninsomniacs.

One other contributing factor that could effect sleep directly is that people with these many distractions tend to get careless about keeping to any kind of sleep routine. They may go to bed and wake up at odd hours, completely throwing off their sleep clock. The effect of this carelessness, as you saw in the first chapter, is that before long their bodies don't know when to go to sleep, and they either end up with insomnia or aggravate the sleeplessness they already have.

There is another part of your sleep profile that is just as important as, or maybe even more important than, how long you sleep or what your particular style of sleep happens to be. That is what time your body clock tells you to sleep. Getting your six or seven or eight hours or more of sleep isn't going to really help you unless you get it at the time of day when it will do you the most good.

This sleep timing is what distinguishes the larks, the early-to-bed-and-early-to-rise sleepers, from the owls, whose idea of early-to-bed might be midnight. No one knows exactly what makes some people larks and others owls; the best guess now is that it is mainly a hereditary trait. Whatever the reason, it's a fact of life that some people hit the bedroom floor with their feet running while others need twenty minutes just to open each eye and stumble out of bed each morning.

We all have a peak of efficiency and activity during the day. For larks this comes in the morning, when they are regular fireballs, knocking off hours of work while the owls around them are still trying to figure out what day it is. At the end of the day, the average lark is burnt out, ready to head back to the nest. By that time, however, the owls are just hitting their stride, taking up where the larks left off. Depending on how the owl's body clock is set, this surge may carry him or her late into the evening.

This peak of activity is a regular, predictable event in every lark and owl's day. It's part of a built-in rhythm that you have moving in you every day. Body rhythm experts have found that they can keep track of these changes simply by following shifts in your body's temperature. Every day your temperature fluctuates one or two degrees. It is low when you get out of bed in the morning and starts to climb as the day wears on. When your temperature is at its peak, so is your alertness.

After the peak, your body is slowly easing itself down toward the level where it is getting ready to go to sleep. As you doze off at night, your body temperature is about a degree lower than it was at its high point during the day. Somewhere in the dead of night, between 3:00 and 4:00 A.M., it hits bottom. People kept awake at that point in their cycle find that their reflexes slow down, they lose muscle coordination, solving simple math problems becomes difficult, and they also feel slightly depressed. It's the part of the day when seriously ill hospital patients suddenly die or when other patients will suddenly have strange overreactions to drugs.

Fortunately for many of us who are larks or larkish, this low is no problem, since it comes during sleep, when we are least affected by it. For the owl, things can get a little more difficult. If you have to be awake at six in the morning, but your body isn't ready to go to sleep until about 1:00 A.M., your rest is really going to suffer. Suppose you decide to go to bed at a reasonable hour, say around 10 P.M. What most likely will happen is that you'll lie in bed waiting for sleep that is really three hours off. What's worse, the next morning you'll find yourself dragging an unwilling body out of bed, a body that still wants to sleep. It may say six o'clock by your alarm clock, but by body time it could be 3:00 A.M., the low point of your day and probably the worst possible time to start work.

For owls, it's a cruel fact of life that it's a lark's world, especially when it comes to jobs. If you want to work and you're a late-night person, you usually end up shoehorning a 12:00-to-8:00 body into a 9:00-to-5:00 job and paying the consequences of having mostly miserable nights of sleep. You know you're going against the grain of one of your most basic body rhythms, but, you may say to yourself, what kind of choice have I got?

Ideally, you could do what one twenty-eight-year-old school teacher did. She was an owl who usually started her first class of the day barely conscious, and even that minimal awareness was the result of three cups of black coffee first thing in the morning. She enjoyed teaching, but the short hours of sleep were grinding her down. Getting up in the morning was pure torture, and going to sleep at an early enough hour proved impossible.

After a while she gave up trying to sleep and, since she needed the extra money anyway, got a job working at a small nightclub. She began to enjoy her part-time job—helping to manage the small club and booking some of the performers—much more, and teaching, less. Finally the club owner offered her a full-time job helping to manage the club. She quit teaching and accepted his offer. "I've never re-gretted it," she now says. "I've always been a night person and the job suits me fine. I sleep better. I now have friends who are awake when I am, and I'm doing something I like."

That is the ideal solution, to find a job that is in tune with your body clock. It's not easy to do unless you have your own business and can change your hours without losing money, or unless you work in the kind of career—freelance writer, artist, or consultant of some kind—where your hours are completely flexible. Also, if you are in a line of work that has around-the-clock shifts—which these days could include anything from nursing to computer programing—you might be able to change to one that suits you best.

This approach has some obvious limitations. First, finding that per-fect job is often easier said than done. (As it is, you may have trouble just hanging on to the one you've got.) The second problem is, even if you do find the right work, switching over to the hours that suit you best may create more problems than it solves. Being a late-night person can put a real strain on a marriage, especially if your spouse happens to be a lark and by nature not sympathetic to your schedule. If you are in this situation, you've probably already had a few arguments about one of you watching late-night movies while the other is trying to sleep, or maybe the trouble one of you has with getting the other up in the morning has been discussed a few times. Taking a job that might keep you away from home at odd hours could just add more pressure to a slightly weakened marriage.

Fortunately there is an alternative that could let you work 9:00-to-5:00 hours and still let you get a decent night's sleep. It's a system of retraining your body clock so that it's more in tune with the day-night cycle. After years of studying and working with people whose body rhythms are out of phase with much of the rest of society, sleep ex-perts at Montefiore Hospital's Sleep-Wake Disorders Unit in New York and at Stanford University figured out a way to reset a person's clock.

They've discovered that going to bed early to get enough sleep is a waste of time. What you have to do instead is push your body clock ahead by one whole day. For some reason, that alone seems to work. The way to do it is by going to bed one hour later on each successive night, while getting the same total number of hours sleep. If you ordinarily go to bed at 2:00 A.M., for example, make your bedtime three o'clock the next night, four o'clock the night after that, and so forth. If you ordinarily sleep eight hours, get up eight hours after your bedtime, whenever it is. It's a time-consuming system, but it usually works.

Some people resist even this drastic recalibration of their inner beat. They may not only have a different sleep-wake schedule of their own, but they may also seem to have a whole different day built into them. Often they aren't running on a twenty-four-hour schedule, but one that's twenty-five hours long or even longer. When people, as part of experiments, shut themselves out from all the time cues of the twenty-four-hour day—such as night and day, definite meal times, the morning ritual of going to work—a natural urge seems to expand the body cycle to a twenty-five-hour day. This could mean that a human is a twenty-five-hour animal gently coerced into following the twenty-four-hour rhythm of the earth's rotation.

The body clocks of some people completely ignore all standard time cues and move according to their own internal rhythms. The blind, who are immune to the time-cue effect of light, are probably the most common examples of this. One Stanford University survey of a group of blind people turned up the fact that over three-fourths complained of sleeping problems that seemed to come and go with a predictable regularity, as though they would periodically come into phase and go out of phase with the regular twenty-four-hour day.

To find out what was going on, a group of sleep experts studied one of the blind who had a particularly rough time sleeping. He was a twenty-eight-year-old student who had been blind from birth and who had recently noticed that he would have regular bouts with insomnia that would run for two or three weeks at a stretch and then disappear. None of the usual treatments was able to bring him back in tune with twenty-four-hour sun time.

After examining him for close to a month, the doctors found the reason why. All of his regular body cycles of temperature, alertness, physical ups and downs, and hormone output were following not a solar day, but a lunar day, which is 24.9 hours long. They also found that there was something familiar about the times he felt sleepy—they coincided with the local times for low tide. None of their efforts to reset his clock succeeded, and so far he is still stubbornly attuned to his personal day.

If you can't bring your body time into line with your work day, don't want to go through marching your bedtime around the clock, and don't want to go hunting for a job that suits your internal schedule, you can do what one patient at Montefiore did. She was a real owl who couldn't seem to bring her body in line with her work schedule. It resisted all efforts to be retrained. She was never able to completely adjust to those sluggish wakeups in the morning, but she got something that helped. She got her dream job, working as an editor on a prestigious national magazine. Getting that position gave her the drive she needed to overcome her morning lethargy. "She still has trouble getting started," said a Montefiore psychologist, "but she can cope. The point is, you can overwhelm lots of your body processes."

Part of the secret of being in control is knowing what there is to control. It's possible, for example, that you are feeling sluggish in the morning because you are sleeping too much. Sleep, and especially dreaming, is hard work for the brain. The reason you don't feel as alert in the morning as you think you should could be because you no longer need the same amount of sleep you customarily get. That morning hangover feeling could be the result of a sleep overdose. By taking the time to figure out what your personal sleep needs are, you might be able to ferret out problems like this.

You probably already have a general idea of what shape your sleep appetite takes if you normally get a good night's rest. How many hours you need will probably range anywhere from five to ten hours, which seem to be the limits of normal sleep. If your sleep time exceeds these limits, you probably deserve to be a footnote in a medical paper. With a little extra effort, you can get a more exact idea of what your personal sleep quotient is. You might be a six-hour-a-night person trying to sleep seven, or a nine-hour-a-night individual trying to get by on eight.

A simple, sloppy way to get your sleep quota is just to let your body tell you when to go to bed and when to wake up. You'll probably have to wait until you take a quiet vacation to do this, since it's better to give your body complete freedom on both ends of the night.

Your body alarm clock may not coincide with the one that gets you up to go to work in the morning. After about a week or so of letting your body run free, add up all your sleep nights and figure out the average time slept. The number you get will give you a rough idea of what your sleep appetite is.

There's also a more exacting way, which is to copy what many sleep clinics do with their insomniac patients and others who have sleep disorders. You can keep a sleep log. This is exactly what it sounds like—a daily record of your sleep habits and any other relevant information. The complexity of sleep diaries varies, and you can make yours as elaborate as you want or as simple; but at the very least the log should note the following five items every day:

- The time you went to bed
- The time you awoke
- How long you think it took you to fall asleep
- The total time you slept
- How you felt the next morning (rested and alert, or fatigued and a little irritable).

Leave your sleep log—which could be a diary, an appointment calendar, or simply a sheet of paper—close by your bed so you can fill it in as soon as you wake in the morning.

If you wish, you can also add a little more information about the periods before and after sleep. For example, you might also note:

- If you had any trouble getting to sleep or staying asleep.
- If you took any pills or had a drink to help you sleep.
- If you had coffee, tea, hot chocolate, or any cola drinks within three or four hours of bedtime.
- How you spent your time just before going to sleep: whether you were working, reading, watching television, exercising, or even napping. A one- or two-word description would be enough.
- At night you might note if you took any naps during the previous day.
- You might also give yourself a general rating of how you felt that past day (alert, or a little tired).

The more information you record, the sharper will be the focus on the kinds of habits that can help or hinder a night's sleep. Too often we absorb into our presleep rituals the cause of our insomnia.

Whatever format you choose, keep daily records for a period of two weeks. At the end of those fourteen nights, add up all the hours you slept and figure out the nightly average. This should give you a good idea of what is a decent night's rest for you. Once you've done this, go back over your log one day at a time. You may get a few surprises. It's typical that the total amount of sleep you get fluctuates from night to night. You may see as much as an hour-and-a-half difference between one night and the next. This is nothing to get very concerned about. No one sleeps exactly the same number of hours every day. These shifts are part of the normal sleep routine.

If you have insomnia, or had it on certain nights, this sleep log may come in handy for providing you with clues about how good or bad your sleep habits are. For example, check and see if you went to bed at approximately the same time every night. Keeping an erratic bedtime schedule is one sure way to throw off your sleep rhythms and keep yourself wide awake and waiting for sleep. Did any other bad habits show up that might cut into your rest? Did you take a sleeping pill or have a nightcap of some kind? These solutions often deliver less than they promise and end up ruining rather than helping sleep, especially if they are nightly habits.

What about other nasty habits? Are you taking too many drugs such as the xanthines? Drinks typically made from xanthines go under the names of coffee, tea, cocoa, and cola. Drinking these too close to bedtime is like taking a wakeup pill. You can also get a similar effect by working right up until bedtime or exercising just before going to bed. Doing work stirs up the mind, and exercise arouses the body—not the best state to be in if you're trying to get some rest.

If you're in the habit of taking a nap every day, your sleep has probably adjusted to this routine. If you take naps sporadically, they might derail your sleep routine so that you end up expecting more sleep than is your due.

Another possible cause of your insomnia that may not show up on your sleep log is a body rhythm that is out of step with your day. This is something you can usually sense in at least a vague way, but if you have any doubts, you can do what some sleep clinics do: take your temperature. As was mentioned before, the well-tuned body doesn't really heat up until the middle of the day. As you get out of bed and get into bed your body should be a little cooler. Sleep experts have found that by doing periodic temperature checks they can approximately chart the ups and downs of your sleep-wake rhythm.

With a little patience you can do the same thing. All you need is an oral thermometer and a total of twenty minutes each day for about a week. The idea is to get an all-day temperature profile of your body from the time you get up to the time you go to sleep at night. Start by taking your temperature in the morning before you get out of bed. Leave the thermometer in your mouth a full five minutes, note the reading carefully, and write it down. Women who are near ovulation should wait until that time has passed, since their body temperatures are naturally higher then. In the course of the day, take two more readings, one at about 11:00 A.M. and a second around 2:00 P.M. Take your last reading once you've lain down in bed and are ready for sleep.

It's important to keep track of each of the four daily recordings and to read the thermometer as precisely as possible. While your basic body temperature does shift, the difference is usually only about one degree, and seldom, if ever, more than two, so you are dealing with a very subtle change.

If your body is in tune, then your temperature highs should come in the daytime. If you're not quite in synchrony with your day, you may find that your temperature reaches a high late in the evening, a sign that you haven't really calmed down enough to go to sleep yet. This technique can't compare with the kind of sophisticated temperature checks that are performed in sleep laboratories, but it should give you some idea of how smoothly your inner tempo is blending with your day.

If you have no trouble sleeping, then what comes out as your average night on your sleep log is your approximate sleep need. Don't worry if it seems too small, if it doesn't seem like enough. The number of hours you sleep each night is not as important as how you feel the next day. And feeling fine is a sign that you are getting the right amount of sleep, whatever the number of hours.

Once you've found the limits of your sleep time, you may decide that you'd like to create a little healthy insomnia of your own and cut back your sleep time by a few minutes or even an hour or so.

After all, most of us could use the extra waking time. If you're extremely busy, a little insomnia does not always have to be a curse. It can add a few more hours to a busy day. The problem with most spells of sleeplessness is that most tend to come when they're least expected and least useful. It would be much more practical if we could control our insomnias to a degree and shrink the time we spend sleeping. Is it possible?

It depends on whom you ask. According to Dr. Ernest Hartmann, scientific evidence gathered so far seems to indicate that most people can probably get by on about six hours' sleep with very little problem. University of Florida scientist Dr. Wilse Webb doesn't exactly agree with this position. If anything, he says, most of us are probably not sleeping enough. Besides, sleep cannot be stretched or squeezed like an accordian. "We can no more wish, demand, or force sleep into different lengths," he has said, "than we can wear a smaller size shoe."

The subject is always good for a polite argument among sleep people because both the pros and the cons can point to one study or another that has succeeded or failed at condensing a person's sleep time. If you were to take a vote today, however, you would likely find that, based on what is known, the pros are in the lead; that is, it looks like some people can cut back on their sleep without suffering any consequences.

The most spectacular example of this was an Australian draftsman named Mr. H., who shared top billing with another short sleeper in a medical report entitled, "Two Cases of Healthy Insomnia." The authors, Henry Jones and Ian Oswald, worked in the Department of Psychiatry at the University of Western Australia, studying sleep and the sleepless. Concerning Mr. H., they wrote, "about six years previously he had decided to give up sleeping much because he was too busy." Mr. H. routinely slept three hours a night and functioned fine during the day. He needed the extra time, he said, because in addition to his job he was also tremendously active in local church and youth organizations. He would take some of the hours he once spent sleeping and stay up working on his organizational paper work.

This ability to live and work comfortably twenty-one hours out of the day appeared to be an inherited gift in Mr. H.'s case. He told Jones and Oswald that his father had been the same way in his younger days. There were nights, he said, when his father didn't bother going to bed at all. Now that his father was older, the man added, he had to sleep a few hours every night.

In the same report, Jones and Oswald mention another patient, a fifty-four-year-old businessman, who never bothered to make a decision about cutting back on his sleep. He was an active and energetic individual who said he managed very easily on three hours' sleep and had done so for the past twenty years. Both men were invited to spend a night in the sleep lab so that the experts could study them. They came in, did a quick three hours, and were gone. Their sleep also had one other feature in common. Shortly after they lay down they dropped almost instantly into the deep, deep levels of stage-3 and stage-4 sleep and stayed there for most of their rest. This seems to be characteristic of every short sleeper whose sleep has been checked in a lab, and it even happens to people who have their sleep reduced to a few hours as part of an experiment. When pressed for time, the body and brain seem to have a craving for the deeper part of non-REM sleep, suggesting that that part of a night's sleep is the most basic and necessary.

These two men had a natural gift for this kind of healthy insomnia, so it was no problem for them to get by on less than half the amount of sleep required by the average person. Although they knew it wasn't realistic to expect that everyone could stretch his or her waking day to twenty-one hours, many sleep experts, intrigued by these extreme cases of short sleepers, wanted to find out just how much sleep could be lopped off a night's rest. What was the least amount of rest the average person could get and still function normally?

One of the better efforts to answer this question was made at the Naval Medical Neuropsychiatric Hospital in San Diego, where three people—two men and a woman—volunteered for a sleep-shrinking experiment. At the start of the test they had sleep times that averaged between seven and one-half and seven and three-quarters hours. The plan was to cut their sleep down to four hours, or as close to it as possible. Each person was put on a sleep diet that required him or her to go to bed a half-hour later every Saturday night. This was scheduled to go on every week for five months or until everyone became too exhausted to continue.

At first the diet went smoothly. Every Saturday the three would stretch out their day by thirty minutes more, usually with no more aftereffect than a slight grogginess the first day or two of the week. As sleep times got shorter, the effects became more noticeable. They began having trouble getting up the next morning and staying awake during the day once past the six-hour mark. Weekly tests of their mood and mental agility began to show that they were bending slightly under the pressure.

The really critical point proved to be the five-hour threshhold. When they reached that point, the effects of short sleep were more obvious. They were oversleeping more and catching naps during the day. One even had a family member hang around with him to make sure he stayed awake the full nineteen hours. One of the volunteers dropped out of the experiment at this point. The naps and over-sleeping got even worse for the other two at the four-and-one-half and four-hour levels. From five hours of sleep on down, the two remaining volunteers registered lows in being tired, depressed, and just plain miserable.

After the test was over, the two people were told to relax and in the months that followed to let their bodies tell them how much sleep they should be getting. For as long as a year later, both people were routinely sleeping an hour to an hour and a half less than usual. They felt perfectly fine and didn't seem to suffer at all from their slightly shorter sleep time.

Before you go off and try the same kind of experiment, you should know that the two people in charge of this sleep diet, Drs. Laverne Johnson and William MacCleod, were careful to point out that it's not as easy as it may have looked. They found that it took a lot of will power to cut down on sleep and stick to the schedule. For that reason, they hand-picked three people who were intensely interested in reducing their nightly sleep and were therefore highly motivated. Even with this high interest, it took the support of friends and the researchers themselves to help the people stay on their low-sleep diet.

Another factor that seemed to help was having a tight and active daily schedule. This provided some of the drive to cut down on sleep and to stick to the routine of stretching out the day. The one person who dropped out of the experiment left shortly after he finished working at a part-time job. When Johnson and MacCleod asked the man why he was leaving, he explained that since he had stopped working "there was nothing to get up for."

The evidence from this and similar experiments is that if you decide to cut down on your sleep, six hours is probably the minimum amount you should try for. Below that level, people start suffering from the shortened hours. They feel "headachey," worn out, are constantly craving sleep, and start to have difficulty concentrating. Before you attempt any kind of sleep reducing, you should first have a realistic idea of approximately how many hours you now sleep. It could be that getting six hours will not be enough for you if, for example, you normally sleep nine. Take about two weeks to keep at least a minimal sleep log so you know about how many hours you have to start with.

Once you've figured out your sleep time, plan a schedule similar to the one used at the naval hospital. Instead of reducing your time every week, give yourself at least two weeks to adjust to each cut. Every other Saturday night, go to bed thirty minutes later than you did in the previous weeks. Saturday night is a good choice because it gives you Sunday to adjust to some of the initial shocks that come with getting a little less sleep. Take at least two weeks to adjust to the shorter schedule and then, if you want to cut back a little more, repeat the Saturday night procedure. You'll know that you have passed your comfortable limit of sleep loss if you feel drowsy much of the time and find yourself fighting the urge to doze off in your quieter moments.

You may find that a thirty-minute cut is too drastic for your body to handle comfortably. If this is the case, try fifteen-minute cutbacks instead. Whatever schedule you choose, you must be faithful to it to retrain your sleep habit. People have shortened their sleep time by as much as two and one-half hours this way, but it is a system that will put your will power to the test.

When you're submitting yourself to this masochistic regimen, it helps to have some kind of motivator to get you out of bed in the morning. You should choose a motivator that suits your nature. Fear works best for some people. One man I know sets his alarm to take his morning shower, shave, dress, and get out of the house. The desire for self-improvement may work for others, such as early morning joggers who slip their feet into icy cold running shoes and go out to do their daily miles. Still others may rely on the lure of that first cup of coffee to get them out of bed. One woman bought a variable timer—

the kind that turns your lights off and on to fool burglars while you're away—and connected it to her electric coffee maker. The timer is set so that the coffee will be brewed just about the time her alarm goes off in the morning. Whatever helps, do it. With a little trial and error, you should be able to come up with your own motivator.

There is a lazy man's alternative to following this Prussian regimen of self-denial: take a nap every day. History has it that Winston Churchill fought the Battle of Britain on four hours' sleep per night and twenty-minute naps in the daytime. People with a habit of napping daily do seem to sleep fewer hours than those who don't nap. In one study of napping, Naval Research Center sleep experts even managed to train a group of people to replace temporarily two nights of sleep with periods of napping during the day. For two days a group of people followed a rigid, round-the-clock schedule of two hours of wake time followed by an hour nap. In a twenty-four-hour day this would give them a full eight hours of sleep parceled out in one-hour bits. Although they felt a little sleepy at first, the nappers settled into the routine with amazing ease. Not only did they sleep less than the time allotted for them, but they did consistently well on various performance tests given during each of their two-hour minidays.

According to body rhythm expert Gay Gaer Luce, author of *Body Time*, one reason why naps work is because they mesh so well with an inner cycle that steadily swings between periods of relaxation and periods of activity. Just as there are steady, predictable periods of REM and non-REM sleep at night, there are alternating periods of alertness and sleepiness during the day. These periods come and go every ninety minutes or so, just as the sleep periods do. People who nap successfully learn to recognize when the periods of relaxation come, and jump in with a nap to take advantage of them. One of the advantages of this habit is that it seems to cut back on how much sleep they need at night.

The later in the day you take a nap, the more likely this is to happen. Studies have found that morning naps give you mostly REM sleep, whereas afternoon naps consist mainly of deep, stage-4 sleep. They also found that while a nap early in the day may leave you refreshed, it may not affect your nightime sleeping at all. If you want to make sure to get the sleep-reducing effect, try to hold off your napping until after four o'clock in the afternoon.

Besides reducing sleep time, napping has another fringe benefit. It sharpens your mind and mood. People who habitually take naps twenty to thirty minutes long are more alert, solve complex math problems more easily, do better on performance tests, and in general are in a much better mood than they were before nap time. Psychologist Frederick Evans of the University of Pennsylvania was so impressed by how well his nap-takers did on tests that he suggested businesses could benefit by providing nap rooms for employees who would prefer to take a sleep break instead of a coffee break.

Just as a practical matter, you may be wondering how you can nap at work, far from the comforts of your bedroom. You can take a tip from professional nappers who, like the 900-pound gorilla in an old joke, sleep anywhere they want—on planes, buses, trains, in cars, or even at or near their desks. I knew one editor who would shut the shades, turn out the lights, and close the door to his office for his daily nap, which he took while lying on the floor. He was in the habit of stretching out in front of his desk, until one day his secretary came in and, not seeing him, accidentally stepped on him. Even napping can be dangerous to your health.

You may find floor space at a premium in your office, or you may prefer not to lie on the floor. In that case, you can rough it at your desk. One woman had her napping down to a science. Every day at 3:30 she'd open her desk drawer, take out a small pillow, set it on the desk in front of her, and, while still sitting in her chair, would lay her head down on it and get a quick twenty winks. Another woman I know, a lawyer, perfected her own sitting-up nap position in which she first crosses her legs, resting them on her bottom desk drawer (pulled out for that purpose), folds her arms across her chest, making sure to tuck her hands under her arms for added warmth, and drops her chin to her chest. And in a few seconds, she's gone.

To get the most out of these short rest periods, there are a few additional facts you should know. First of all, closing your eyes and resting for twenty minutes is not napping, and won't bring you any of napping's benefits. You actually have to go to sleep to achieve the alert, refreshed state of mind described earlier. Secondly, you will benefit more from naps if you make them a daily habit. You may or may not have problems doing this. There are some people who seem to be natural nappers. They can turn on sleep the way the rest of us flick a light switch. No one has proved that this is an ability that is inherited, but so far the evidence is that some people are better at it than others. The only way you can find out if you're a napper or non-napper is by giving it a try for a week or two. Don't expect to be invigorated by just one nap taken every once in a while. If you've ever done it, you probably already are acquainted with the typical results: you wake in a stupor, with a stale taste in your mouth, and your mind seems frozen in a permanent fog. It's only when the nap becomes a regular fixture in your day that you can expect to get any benefit from it.

Lastly, if you have insomnia, forget everything that's been said about napping. Grabbing snatches of sleep during the day won't do anything for your sleep problem, and is likely to make it worse. Insomniacs have a hard enough time getting the sleep they need without napping.

Why do you need any sleep at all? Why worry about how much sleep you need? You know that you feel more alert and in better shape, both physically and psychologically, after a good night's sleep. You've known that all your life. But what exactly does sleep do for you? For a more sophisticated, scientific answer, we have to look to an expert like psychologist Dr. Allan Rechtschaffen of the University of Chicago, who says, "I feel better after sleeping, but why? I don't know, and nobody else does either." And he's right. You can go through the volumes of papers and books written by sleep researchers in the past twenty-five years and you'll find basically the same answer. "From a strictly neurological and physiological viewpoint, there is no objective proof that any restorative or recuperative process gets underway," says one psychologist. Or, according to another professional sleep watcher, "Need is a very strange term when applied to sleep. We know we need food because if we don't get it, we will die. It isn't clear what sleep will do for us." You can take some comfort in the fact that, right now, your opinion about what sleep does for you is as good as any expert's.

It is fairly clear that, whatever the reason, we do need sleep. Our bodies tell us that every night. But what happens if we ignore those sleep signals and keep on going? As was mentioned in the first chapter, animal experiments based on doing this produced drastic results—psychotic behavior and even death. Tentative tests with people seemed to confirm some of these findings and to support a popular theory on sleep. That theory held that dreams act as a kind of psychological safety valve, letting us work out in nightly fantasies all the anxieties and hostility that we repress during the day. Take away the dreams, the experts figured, and you take away this safety valve. As a result, you'd be bottling up all these repressed feelings and putting a real strain on the mind. If allowed to build up enough, these feelings would work themselves out in strange, possibly psychotic behavior.

In one test a man was given amphetamines which blanked out his REM sleep (the time when most dreams occur) for fourteen nights. At the beginning of the study he was a tight-lipped teetotaler, somewhat on the prudish side. After about two weeks without REM sleep, he turned into an obnoxious loudmouth. One night he said he wanted to go to a bar and see a strip show. Another time he was caught trying to cheat a waitress.

Experiments in wiping out sleep completely have produced a few odd physical reactions as well. After about two and a half days without sleep one group of men tested started feeling sick to their stomachs, had sore, aching joints, developed nervous twitches in their eyeballs, and had hand tremors as well.

All these omens of insanity and physical decay, as it turned out, were highly overrated. What helped to defuse them was a seventeen-year-old boy and his science fair project. In 1964 a San Diego high-school student named Randy Gardner decided that as his project he would try to break the world record for staying awake. At that time, according to the *Guinness Book of World Records*, the record was 260 hours (10 days, 20 hours). Randy enlisted two classmates to keep him awake and act as official witnesses to history.

He had already logged about eighty hours awake when Dr. William Dement of Stanford University and Dr. Laverne Johnson of the San Diego Naval Hospital joined Randy's experiment to offer a little medical expertise and also to observe him. After 11 days—264 hours— Randy decided to finally go to sleep. What was amazing about his record-breaking 264-hour day was that it had no serious physical or psychological effect on him while he was awake. Equally surprising was the short amount of sleep he needed to make up for those eleven lost nights. After only fourteen hours' sleep he woke completely rested.

The following night and every night after that he returned to a normal sleep time of about eight hours.

Studies and experiences like these help tell us what sleep doesn't do if we lose it—it won't kill us or drive us crazy—but so far they haven't given us any definite answers concerning what it does do. In cases like this, where the experts have no answers, they come up with the next best thing, theories. Right now there are two major theories. The first is the restorative theory, which views sleeping as maintenance time for the body and brain. The second is called the adaptive behavioral theory, which essentially explains sleep as a survival habit that we picked up back in prehistoric days.

Sleep clinicians who favor the restorative theory point out that each of the two kinds of sleep seem to serve a special purpose. Non-REM sleep seems to be necessary for keeping the body in shape with nightly repairs. Researchers know, for example, that growth hormone, absolutely necessary for a child's normal development, is pulsed into the bloodstream in its greatest amounts during stage-4 sleep. Dr. Ernest Hartmann of the Boston State Hospital's Sleep Laboratory points out that sleep tests showed individuals need more stage-3 and stage-4 sleep after heavy physical work or exercise, as do people on starvation diets and even recently circumcised infants. On the other hand, individuals who were selectively starved of non-REM sleep complained of stiff, aching muscles and joints the morning after.

REM sleep seems to be brain sleep. People deprived of REM sleep find that their memory suffers. In one experiment at the University of Colorado, people who went to sleep after a memory test had better recall than those who didn't sleep. Retarded children and adults who have suffered brain damage through a stroke or injury and are unable to speak also have less REM sleep than would be normal for them. Hartmann also believes that the brain uses REM-sleep time to reprogram its circuits of nerve cells with the new information that it has stored during the day. Some believe part of this programing recharges that part of the brain which controls our urges and impulses. Without REM sleep, people might lose all social inhibitions, like the man who wanted to go to a strip show and cheat a waitress.

Other researchers, such as Dr. Wilse Webb of the University of Florida, claim that sleep is a survival habit carried over from primitive times when humans really had a reason to be afraid of the dark. With no ability to function in the pitch black of night, early humans were better off staying at home in the safety of their caves. And that's what sleep forced them to do. This behavior-control part of sleep became a built-in mechanism that has stayed with us till this day, even though we have conquered the night with electric lights.

Those who believe this adaptive behavior theory point out that the claim that sleep helps restore the body may make good common sense, but it doesn't make good scientific sense. If a night's sleep were so important to putting the body back in shape, then losing part or all of a night's sleep should do much more damage to us than it seems to. According to the restorative theory, Randy Gardner should not have survived his eleven days without sleep with as little trouble as he had.

Another intriguing fact, pointed out by Dr. Webb, is that each animal's sleep is peculiarly suited to promoting its survival. Predators generally sleep longer than their prey, who stand to benefit by staying awake and alert much more of the time. While gazelle sleep for a few hours each day, their enemy the lion may get as much as sixteen hours of rest. Sleep also suits feeding habits. The elephant only gets four hours of sleep because it needs the twenty hours to find the 400 to 600 pounds of greenery it eats in the average day.

Theories like these may make interesting topics for conversation, but understanding the purpose of sleep doesn't help when you're not getting any. By finding out how much sleep you need you may gain some insight into your insomnia or even discover that you don't have a sleep problem after all. Or, you may find that your sleep problem is very real and very persistent, wrecking your nights and making you miserable during the day as well. If your insomnia doesn't go away in a few weeks and it really bothers you, most likely you'll end up seeking help from your doctor. And if he or she can't help you, then it's time for the ultimate weapon against insomnia—the sleep clinic.

3.
A Night
at the Laboratory

"There she goes again." The technician pointed to the two robot pens making up-and-down scribbles on the seemingly endless sheet of graph paper rolling underneath them. It would happen over and over again, two or three times a minute. The pens would be still, their tips lightly trailing a thin line of black ink on the moving paper, and then suddenly would explode into a frenzy of scribbling for a second or two, then just as suddenly stop.

It was nearly midnight. We were standing in the brightly lit equipment room of the Sleep Clinic at the Dartmouth Medical School, watching another person's sleep being monitored and charted for us by the polygraph machine, probably the single most valuable piece of equipment in any sleep laboratory. Its job is to monitor the body and brain of the person sleeping and translate what it finds into a cryptic, machine shorthand that, on a sheet of recording paper, looks like rows of wavy lines, scribblings, and large and small jagged waves. Every second of a night's sleep is recorded this way. By morning, the notes the machine is taking will fill a sheet of paper about two feet wide and a thousand feet long.

On the other side of the wall from us, in one of the clinic's small but comfortable bedrooms, slept the woman the polygraph was watching. Incredibly, she seemed oblivious to the tentacles of thin, electrode-tipped wires taped to the sides of her head, face, and the lower part of her legs as she drifted along in what for her was a normal night's sleep. But as she well knew, it was not a good night's sleep. For years she had been waking each morning feeling worn out and exhausted. She seemed to get very little sleep in spite of the fact that she was convinced she spent the whole night resting quietly. She went from doctor to doctor, from pill to pill, and from one therapy to another in an effort to get a decent night's sleep. Nothing worked, and so she had now turned to the insomniac's last resort, the sleep clinic.

Psychological tests turned up the fact that she was suffering from depression, in itself a common enough cause of insomnia. But her three nights in the laboratory revealed another problem.

"Nocturnal myoclonus, leg twitches," the technician explained, pointing to the frantic burst of scribbling we were watching. Periodically the woman's leg muscles would jerk uncontrollably and, for the space of a second or two, wake her up. The wakeup wasn't long enough for her to recall, but it was enough to interrupt the flow of her sleep. This happened routinely, two or three times a minute, during the first few hours of sleep. Each time it did, the electrodes taped to her leg relayed the movement to the recording pens of the polygraph.

Although there is no perfect cure for this ailment, many people have been able to subdue these leg motions by taking a mild tranquilizer called diazepam, better known as Valium. As is the case with so many serious, long-lasting insomnias, this woman's sleep problem was not so simple that a pill would wipe it out. Her depression was a complicating factor. It would take a thorough study of the 3,000 feet of sleep records generated during her nights at the lab, as well as the information and insights gleaned from psychological tests and interviews with the woman, before her doctor could decide on an effective strategy for attacking her sleep problem. This would be done by Dr. Peter Hauri.

The head of the Dartmouth Sleep Clinic, Dr. Hauri is in many ways typical of those who are members of the small but growing scientific elite of sleep researchers. His speciality is clinical psychology, but to be a competent sleep researcher he has also had to acquire more than a passing familiarity with general medicine, endocrinology, neurochemistry, neurology, otolaryngology, cardiology, psychiatry, and, because of the exotic equipment he sometimes uses, electronics as well. He earned his doctorate at the University of Chicago, as famous for turning out sleep experts as West Point is for generals. And, like most of his colleagues, he divides his time between researching sleep disorders and treating them.

"About two-thirds of the people I see are insomniacs," he told me in his office the morning after we stayed up all night watching the polygraph perform. "In the cases that have come here, the insomnia has run anywhere between two years and a lifetime. Some people have come in here and said 'If you'd only been here forty years ago I would have been able to sleep.' "

Again like most of his colleagues, Dr. Hauri wants to restrict the facilities of the sleep laboratory to treat the most severe cases of chronic insomnia. For that reason, he has a fixed procedure for accepting a new patient that is a little stricter than most laboratories. Because of the clinic's somewhat remote location in the small (population 6,000) town of Hanover in the middle of New Hampshire, and its limited three-bed facilities, Dr. Hauri only accepts for treatment those people he thinks will benefit the most.

All his patients are referred to the sleep lab by their doctors. If you were to write asking for an appointment yourself, he would send you a brochure on the sleep lab and a form letter telling you what to get from your doctor. "That cuts out many referrals already," says Dr. Hauri, "because the doctor may think it's of no use to send them."

If the doctor does think a sleep lab is worth the patient's time and money, he or she sends on information about the patient. Dr. Hauri in turn mails off what he describes as a "miserable package" of questionnaires and forms for the patient to complete. The forms are used to get a psychological profile of the person, his or her sleep habits, and, by using a sleep log, how much sleep the person thinks he or she is getting. "This takes about three or four hours to fill out," explains Dr. Hauri. "At this point some patients quit. I am consciously making it somewhat difficult to come here, in order to weed out, as much as possible, anyone without a serious problem."

What qualifies as a serious problem? An insomnia so bad that it makes you willing to spend four hours filling out a battery of forms and questionnaires. According to Dr. Hauri, chronic insomnia takes a while to surface. You may suffer in silence for as long as six months before you go to a doctor for help. The doctor's treatment typically will be a sleeping pill prescription. That pill works for a few weeks but eventually loses its punch. You go back. The doctor gives you another pill, or a stronger dose of the one you had. That works for a little while longer but soon loses its power as well. You go back again, but the doctor by now has run out of prescriptions. The next thing you know, you're spending four hours filling out Dr. Hauri's miserable package.

Some people never have to go beyond this initial screening point. After examining the package of information, Dr. Hauri may find the person doesn't need to come to his laboratory. It may be that the insomnia is the result of a mild depression that can be treated with an antidepressant or that the insomnia is not as serious as the patient may think. "She may sleep eight hours and think she needs ten," he offers as an example. "She feels okay during the day, but still is a little anxious. She really doesn't have much of an insomnia."

"If I cannot decide what's wrong with the patient," he adds, "the next step is to come to the lab and sleep three nights." On each of these nights the patient reports to the lab about an hour or so before bedtime, to be wired up for a night of sleep. If you should get this far in the sleep clinic treatment, what will happen is that electrode-tipped wires will be taped to areas of your head and other parts of your body so the polygraph machine can keep an all-night record of not only how much you sleep but how good your sleep is as well.

Just how many electrodes you will wear to bed will depend on what kind of sleep problem you have, but at the very least there will be recordings made of your brain waves, muscle tension, and eye movement (one of the key signs of REM sleep). Four electrodes, two on either side of your head on the top and two more at the base of your ear, will pick up changes in your brain waves as you sleep. Two other electrodes, taped near the outside corner of each eye, monitor eye movement, and two taped to your chin are for keeping a record of muscle tension.

Each electrode has a color-coded wire attached to it, and each is meticulously applied by a trained technician. Every spot where an electrode will be attached is first cleansed with alcohol. The electrode gets a dab of sodium chloride jelly to improve the electrical contact with the skin and is then fixed in position with a few strips of translucent tape. As a further precaution, the head is wrapped in layers of white gauze to hold wires and electrodes in place.

Besides these connections, you may also have electrodes attached to your legs to monitor leg twitches and a single electrode in the middle of your back to record your heart rate. You also may have a wire with a temperature-sensitive tip, called a thermistor, placed under your right nostril to record breathing, or under your arm to monitor body temperature.

After being hooked up for the night, you will be led to your bedroom, where each of the wires dangling from you will be plugged into a special terminal, your link with the mechanical sleep-watcher, the polygraph machine. Next to the bed is an intercom to keep you in touch with the scientists in the next room should any problem arise (such as the need to be unplugged so you can go to the bathroom).

As uncomfortable as this all sounds, few people ever have any serious trouble getting to sleep. In fact there is a peculiar problem some insomniacs have called the first-night effect by which they may get one of the best night's sleeps they ever had. Dr. Hauri says that the first night is usually an excellent one in part because the insomniac is looking forward to a poor sleep and is not anxious about it. "It's a matter of 'For twenty years nobody has taken me seriously. Now I can show the whole world how miserably I sleep. I don't mind if I don't sleep all night,' " Dr. Hauri explained.

However good or bad the sleep is, by morning it's all copied down as rows of scrawled lines, each of which has something important to say about your night. Someone like Dr. Hauri who is skilled in reading the language of the sleep recording, called a polysomnogram, can tell by studying these lines how much sleep you got; how deep it was; how many REM dream phases you had; whether you had a restless sleep filled with awakenings and tossing and turning; and how tense you were before and during sleep. He may also spot special problems, such as breath-stopping sleep apnea, leg twitches, or a body rhythm out of phase with the day.

The one part of the sleep record that most clearly charts your movement through the different stages and phases of sleep is the electroencephalogram, or EEG, which measures your brain waves.

Each part of your sleep has a certain brain-wave signature that sets it off from other parts of the night. Even your waking hours look different. When you're alert and awake, your brain waves have an active, ragged look to them, but as you become more relaxed (e.g., just before sleep), your brain starts producing alpha waves, a settled, even series of brain waves.

The waves loosen up a little more in stage-1 sleep, and in stage 2 a different pattern surfaces. The waves stay relaxed and even, but every so often they explode into clusters of high-intensity outbursts called spindles, because that's what they resemble, tightly wound bundles of wire lying on their sides. In stages 3 and especially 4 the waves exhibit their most relaxed patterns, with extravagant Mt. Everest peaks and Grand Canyon valleys drawn in lazy up-and-down sweeps. When REM sleep comes, it brings with it another style of brain wave which looks very much like the wave of an active and alert mind. If you cross-check this with other parts of the recording—the one for muscle tone, for example—you'll find that, while the brain is in a frenzy, the body is as limp as a wet rag.

The sleep record tells only part of the story of a night's sleep. It describes events and changes that can be detected outside of you. The inside story—that is, whether it felt like a good night's rest—has to come from you. For that reason Dr. Hauri has his patients fill out a sleep evaluation form when they get up. After the first night's sleep, he also conducts neurological tests and a detailed interview with the patient. These help him to zero in on the principal cause or causes of the insomnia and to decide on the best treatment for them.

Although the causes of insomnia are conveniently grouped into physical, psychological, and behavioral categories, they don't always come that neatly packaged in real life. An insomnia can be the result of a chain-reaction of causes. For example, the stress of a new job, with its new responsibilities and new worries, may keep you up at night. Finally, when you can stand it no more, you get some sleeping pills from your doctor. The pills become a nightly habit, but in the meantime you have adjusted to the pressures at work. All of a sudden you find you have a new problem: you can't sleep with the pills and you can't sleep without them. What began as a psychological problem is now a drug problem.

The purpose of all the tests, night recordings, and the interview is to sort through the possible causes of your sleeplessness and find which is yours. Finding the correct cause can be a real challenge to a sleep expert's experience, knowledge, and skills. It may sometimes entail a frustrating search through a series of false leads to get at what is the root of the insomnia. "I might find low self-esteem in my psychological tests, or high muscle tension with my behavioral tests, or signs of disruption in the body rhythm," explains Dr. Hauri, "but I might not be personally convinced I'm on the right track."

At these times his instincts often prove to be his most valuable diagnostic tool. In one puzzling case he spent over four hours of interview time talking to a female patient trying to get some sense of what might be behind her sleeplessness. A relaxed, friendly man with an open, almost boyish face, Dr. Hauri bided his time, depending on his skills and training as a psychotherapist to guide him in knowing when to let her talk and when to ask a probing question or two.

"After we had gotten to know each other and when she was somewhat more relaxed, it came out that her problem was that she had a malformed child," he recalls. "When she was pregnant she had used a fair amount of sleep drugs and, even though everyone told her to the contrary, she felt that the drugs had caused the malformations. And when she sleeps at night, these malformations are what she sees."

"She was poised, knew all the right things to say—'Yes I do have a malformed child but those are the breaks.' The cause of her insomnia was very well defended," Hauri adds.

By his own estimate, Dr. Hauri says that slightly more than a third of the insomniacs he sees turn out to have some psychological cause at the root of their sleep problem. About a sixth of the insomnias have medical causes, such as the leg twitches suffered by the woman mentioned at the beginning of this chapter, heavy use of sleeping pills, or any of a number of other reasons ranging from sleep apnea to going through late-night nicotine withdrawal. Finally, about half the insomniacs he sees have trouble sleeping for a number of vague, sometimes unknown reasons. In some instances the problems are behavioral—involving bad bedtime habits or association of insomnia with the bedroom. There are those who wake up at the beginning of every REM dream phase, and those who try to sleep more than they need too. Mixed in are a mystery group of insomniacs who seem to sleep even in an alert state of mind, or who have inexplicable shifts in brain-wave patterns, such as alpha-wave pollution, for example. And they all, at least for the moment, have no scientific explanation or cure.

When he has fixed on what looks like the cause of the sleep problem, Dr. Hauri sends his findings to both doctor and patient, telling them what he's found and listing some recommended treatments to try. Nine months later, he sends off a sleep log to the patient and a letter to the doctor to find out how well the patient did. "My batting average on this nine-month follow-up is that I help three out of four," he says.

The odds are about the same—and so is the elaborate screening process—at just about any sleep clinic you may visit. The major difference between the Dartmouth clinic and one located in or near a big city is often just a matter of size. At Montefiore Hospital's Sleep-Wake Disorders Clinic in New York City, for example, a fifteen-person staff with specialties in cardiology, neurology, psychology, and nose-and-throat medicine works full time handling the large load of patients that come to the clinic each year. Getting in at Montefiore is not quite as difficult as being accepted at the Dartmouth Clinic, and people can apply for treatment there without a doctor's referral. About half the people treated at Montefiore enter on this basis. Before they ever show up at the clinic, they are sent a sleep log to keep track of their sleep for two weeks. As is the case at Dartmouth, some people never make it to the clinic. Just the act of keeping track of their sleep is often enough to convince them that they're sleeping fine. "They actually make appointments and then break them after doing the sleep log," says Montefiore's codirector, Dr. Charles Pollok. "When we call them up to ask why, they say, 'You know, I'm sleeping better now that I see how much rest I have.' "

If you should be one of the unfortunates for whom the sleep log is no help, the next step is to come in for a physical exam, usually given by a staff neurologist. You will also take a battery of psychological tests and go through an interview with a staff psychologist. Based on the information that comes out of these tests, some kind of treatment may be prescribed for you, or you may go on to the next stage of treatment, two nights in the sleep laboratory.

The laboratory setup is essentially the same as the one used at Dartmouth—a polygraph recording information from wires attached to your sleeping body—with one extra bit of technology. The clinic also has a videotape recorder installed in the bedroom where you stay to record your sleep movements. The following morning, you're asked to rate how well you slept, and how you feel. Some clinics, like Montefiore, do this with a number-coded sleep scale. Numbers from one to seven are used for rating states from total alertness to being on the verge of sleep. The number scale is as follows:

1. feeling active
2. functioning at a high level but not at a peak
3. relaxed, awake but not fully alert
4. a little foggy
5. foggy, slowed down
6. sleepy, woozy
7. almost in reveries, cannot stay awake

Everything you've answered on your psychological tests, in your psychological interview, and in your morning-after sleep rating, as well as facts from your sleep past, physical exam, and sleep recordings form the raw material of your diagnosis. A conference of the clinic's experts will be convened and, using their collective expertise in psychology, psychiatry, neurology, and other specialities that apply, will come up with a diagnosis and a plan of action.

"This unit was established as a collaboration between neurology and psychiatry," explained Dr. Pollok, himself a neurologist. "That meant neurologists and psychiatrists would be seeing the patient, sitting around the conference table, and fighting it out on each case. Things got pretty heated up at times, but by and large we found we ended up agreeing on most patients, and we also learned a lot from each other."

The payoff of this learning is a better night's sleep for you. While he doesn't give any batting averages for Montefiore's success in treating insomnia, Dr. Pollok does say that one of the two big surprises the clinic had when it started in 1975 was that even with an imperfect understanding of all the possible causes of insomnia, the clinic was able to take care of most cases with little trouble. The other surprise was the number of insomniacs. The clinic expected most, if not all, of its patients to have trouble sleeping. As it happens, somewhere between one-half and two-thirds of them have trouble sleeping. The rest have trouble staying awake—that is, problems of sleepiness caused by narcolepsy or the breathing defect of sleep apnea.

It's just as well that the tens of millions of the sleepless don't decide to go to a sleep clinic, because even now there are not all that many around. As recently as 1972 there were only four or five sleep clinics in the country. Now, as knowledge about sleep has grown and the ability to diagnose and treat sleep problems has improved, sleep clinics have become more common. But the numbers are still not huge. At last count, there were a little over two dozen sleep clinics in the United States (a state-by-state listing appears on pages 168–173) each with a long waiting list of sleepless or sleepy patients.

How will you know if you should join one of these waiting lines? This is one instance in medicine where patients have as big a say in their diagnosis as their doctors do. Only you know how badly your insomnia affects you. Only you can make the final decision that it is serious enough to justify your going to an expert for help. In general, says Montefiore's Dr. Pollok, you can consider your insomnia serious if you've had trouble getting to sleep or staying asleep on a nightly or almost nightly basis for two months or more. That, he says, is a reasonable standard for gauging just how bad your problem is.

If you feel that your insomnia is getting bad and interfering with your days, your first step should be to go to your family doctor for help. While getting medications such as mild tranquilizers or anti-depressants can help, just visiting the doctor and talking about your sleep problem may be all the cure you need. When nothing the doctor recommends works, and your insomnia stays the same or gets worse, that's the time to go to a sleep clinic.

As you've already seen, specific procedures will vary from one place to another, but in general you will go through some kind of screening process that usually involves sleep logs and psychological and physical tests first. Since you may not have to go on to sleep in the laboratory, there is usually a separate fee for the initial evaluation. At Montefiore, for example, the charge is $150. If you should have to sleep in the laboratory, you may spend anywhere from two to four nights there, depending on that clinic's policy. Costs vary as well, from $200 to $300 a night. (Those figures alone may help you decide your insomnia isn't so bad after all.) Since just about every sleep clinic has approximately the same batting average as Dr. Peter Hauri's, the odds are in favor of your getting your money's worth.

Probably the most succinct and practical guidelines you could ask for in helping to make your sleep clinic decision are these offered by Dr. Hauri: "when nothing works, when your doctor has given up, when you are really slowing down, when you feel you could function so much better if you could get a night's sleep, and if you have the necessary dough," then, he says, it's time to go.

Part of the reason for the expense is that treatment usually has to be customized to your sleep problem. No two insomnias are exactly alike. For that reason, there is no magic formula or miracle pill that will work for all of them. About the only things the chronic insomniacs that Montefiore treats have in common, according to Dr. Pollok, are that they've had their sleep problem for years, that it bothers them practically every night, and that their main complaints are not that they're having trouble falling asleep, but that they keep waking up during the night or early in the morning. "The typical insomniac has trouble with everything," he says. "It's a mixed bag of difficulties."

After you've gone through the screening and have had recordings of your sleep scribbled out by the polygraph, the sleep clinician will first look to see if there is any physical cause for your insomnia. If there is, treatment may be nothing more than referring you to the right specialist if, for example, it turns out your poor sleep is the result of an ulcer condition, nightly migraines, heart pain, a thyroid condition, or any of a number of other problems that could interfere with sleep.

For the more subtle causes, the sleep expert will pick up your sleep recording and start reading it closely. After recording thousands of sleepers, both healthy and unhealthy, sleep experts now know exactly what a normal night's sleep should look like for sleepers of every age. However long or short a healthy person's sleep is, it always follows a known, predictable pattern, first moving down through the stages of non-REM sleep, back up to REM sleep, and then back into non-REM sleep to start the cycle all over again. This is the quality yardstick used to measure every night of recorded sleep.

It sometimes happens that the recording will show that what at first seems to be abnormal is actually perfectly fine. Dr. Hauri tells of one clinic patient, a fifty-one-year-old physics professor who worried because he had to spend at least fourteen hours per day sleeping.

Resting any fewer hours—he once tried cutting back to twelve hours —left him worn out. A few nights in the lab showed that his rest was perfectly normal—for him. He just happened to be one of those rare people who genuinely need fourteen hours of sleep.

When there are real physical problems, they usually do surface in the sleep record. Sleep experts are conditioned to look for the bizarre as well as the ordinary in sleep because they often find it. One patient came to the Montefiore Clinic complaining he wasn't getting enough sleep. He kept dozing off while watching porno films he reviewed for his sex magazine, and at night he snored so loudly his wife made him sleep in another room. A night in the laboratory confirmed the experts' suspicions. He had the potentially dangerous problem of sleep apnea. Throughout his night's sleep he would stop breathing for as long as a minute, wake up gasping for air, and fall back to sleep with a loud snore.

Because his problem was with his windpipe—it kept collapsing during sleep—the doctors cured his insomnia by giving him a second windpipe for sleeping. As part of a routine tracheotomy, surgeons inserted a plastic tube in his neck, leaving a small opening that is sealed up with a small plug during the day. At night when he wants to go to sleep, all the man has to do is unplug his throat and he is able to breathe normally for a satisfying, snore-free night.

The man gained a lot more than a night's sleep from this cure. It saved him from a possible heart attack. Sleep apnea is often seen in people, mostly men, who have heart trouble. Since high blood pressure is one of the side effects of this breath stoppage, it could strain a weak or ailing heart to the point of cardiac arrest. And it saved his marriage as well. With the snoring stopped, he was back in the bedroom and his wife's good graces.

Other physical problems the clinic is particularly adept at finding with the help of the sleep record include the automatic, uncontrollable leg twitching of nocturnal myoclonus, a body clock that is out of synchrony with the twenty-four-hour cycle of night and day, and sleep damage from drugs.

In every case the cure will be customized to your particular case. With one businessman whose leg-twitching problem was ruining both his sleep and his import-export business, the Montefiore experts did not use drugs, but instead helped him sleep "around" the problem.

They found that by helping him push his bedtime up to four in the morning he was able to sleep quietly without the myoclonus problem. With his new bedtime he got up at noon and was at work by 1:00 P.M., a much better rested man.

One thing the sleep doctors will want to know is whether or not you are taking sleeping pills or any other drug, such as alcohol, to help you sleep. The reasons are simple enough. Even when the pills are working, they give you a kind of semisleep, one that is basically a deep stupor with no REM sleep at all. Alcohol has the same effect. What happens over a period of time is that, unless you continue raising the dosage, you are going to lose the knockout power of the pill and just be left with its side effect—a feeble night's sleep. In recording the sleep of one heavy pill-user, Dartmouth's Dr. Hauri found that the patient, a woman in her fifties who had been suffering from insomnia for thirty years, had *no* normal sleep. Not only was she completely missing her nightly quota of REM sleep, but she had none of the deeper stages of non-REM sleep either.

In cases like this, the clinic has to wean both your body and your mind from the habit of taking pills before it can restore you to a normal night's sleep. Depending on the kind of sleeping pill you've been taking, how long you've been taking it, and the size of the dosage, this process can take weeks or, in the most extreme cases, can go on for years. So if you are now taking pills for your insomnia but plan to go to a sleep clinic for a cure for your sleeplessness, be prepared to give them up. No matter how much you may think you need your sleep drugs, the evidence is overwhelming that you are better off without them.

The same applies to alcohol, which not only has the same corrosive effect on your sleep but may lead to alcoholism. You can expect to be told to get out of the habit of having a nightcap of some kind to help you sleep at night. Insomnia is among the many problems that a drink won't cure.

The sleep experts may also want to know about what daytime drugs you are taking. Amphetamine-based diet pills, doses of antihistamines taken for allergies, decongestants used in cold medicines, and some antidepressants such as Dexedrine and Ritalin, can all be anti-sleep and can leave their mark on your sleep recording by wiping out parts of your sleep. It's even possible you may suffer insomnia as a kind of allergic reaction to other drugs as well. There is a case on record of one woman who came to a sleep clinic for help with an insomnia that had been bothering her since she switched back to day work after a three-month stint on a night shift. At first the cause of her sleep problem seemed obvious: she was just having trouble readjusting to her day schedule. After therapy for that did nothing at all, she was asked to come back to the clinic. Another interview revealed that she had recently started taking a birth control pill. At the sleep clinician's suggestion, she stopped taking the pill. Within a week her insomnia evaporated.

Eliminating drug interference with sleep may be all that's necessary to take care of your insomnia, but there may be other complicating factors that turn up once the pill has gone. Psychological causes, of which depression is probably the most common, may be at the root of your insomnia. Some researchers have found that the sleeplessness is a kind of smokescreen for depression, especially in older patients. Some people feel that admitting to being depressed is tantamount to branding themselves as social failures, individuals who can't cope. For them it may be much easier not to confront their depression, but to adopt instead the much more vague complaint of not being able to sleep.

Because of the varieties of depression, no one therapy works all the time. Sleep clinicians may try whatever seems appropriate to the occasion. Some depressions that appear as reactions to a personal tragedy of some kind, such as the death or serious illness of someone close, are called reactive depressions. They respond well to psychotherapy which helps the insomniac weather the life crisis.

A more serious brand of depression is called endogenous because it seems to arise spontaneously from within the person. It has no definite cause. People suffering from this problem typically complain of the bleak, desolate feelings that come with each of a series of awakenings during the night and in the early morning. One treatment that works well in many of these cases is prescribing antidepressants as sleep aids to be taken just before bedtime.

With any psychological problem, treatment may be on a trial-and-error basis, with mixing and matching of different therapies and drugs until the one that works best is found. One of the problems in sorting out psychological problems connected with long-term insomnia is what Dr. Hauri labels the "chicken-or-the-egg" dilemma of cause and effect. Long-lasting insomnia usually brings with it symptoms of depression. Many times it is difficult to tell whether it's the insomnia that has brought on the depression or if it was the other way around. Depression can do its share of ruining your sleep once you get caught up in the vicious cycle of being-depressed-about-losing-sleep and losing-sleep-about-being-depressed. Whether it is always the depression that sets the cycle rolling, no one is sure.

In experiments where normal sleepers are deliberately deprived of sleep, researchers have found one of the side effects of this induced insomnia is a depressed mood. If the insomnia lasts long enough, this depression it sets off could become a fixture in your personality. "After ten years of lousy sleep," says Dr. Hauri, "even the best of us might get worn down." The only way sleep experts could ever know for sure which came first is by doing an experiment that for ethical reasons will never be done: a group of normal people would have to be turned into permanent insomniacs by some Dr. Frankenstein technique and then watched to see what happens.

If your insomnia turns out to be the product of a deeply rooted bad habit—a behavioral insomnia—the tactic the sleep lab will use against it will be to have you develop some kind of good habit. For example, if it looks like you're careless about when you go to bed, they might give you a strict bedtime schedule to follow and a sleep log to fill out. They may even redesign your bedtime ritual so that the bedroom will no longer be the threatening black hole of insomnia it now seems to be. After years of experience with this problem, sleep clinicians now have a small arsenal of training techniques (see Chapter 5) they can turn to. These may include everything from special antiinsomnia strategies that get you out of the bedroom when you can't sleep to a variety of presleep habits ranging from afternoon exercise to various mind games.

Special relaxation techniques, treated in detail in Chapter 6, also seem to help counteract the dread that comes with lying in bed tensely waiting for sleep. You might be given instructions on muscle tension-and-release exercises, or variants of transcendental meditation, if that seems to work for you, or some kind of biofeedback where you learn to pick up subtle cues from your body that help you relax it. The sleep clinicians will probably have you try a series of techniques until you find the one that works best for you.

It may turn out that your sleep problem is a body clock out of step with your daily schedule. Temperature readings taken during your nights in the sleep laboratory should provide some clue to how well your sleep cycle meshes with the day-night cycle. A temperature that is climbing, not diving, at bedtime is one sign your body is following a different drummer. The first thing the sleep experts will try to do is put you back on the track with your day. Sometimes this doesn't take any more than holding you to a strict bedtime schedule. In more stubborn cases, they might try to tease the sleep part of your sleep-wake cycle into position by walking it around the clock, bumping up your bedtime an hour each day (the technique described in Chapter 2). If that doesn't work, you might be told to try and get a job that suits your schedule.

Dr. Hauri had one patient who had been fired from her job because her body clock worked against her getting up early enough to get to work on time. Once she was unemployed, her time was her own, and so he told her to follow her own sleep-wake urges and keep a sleep log on her natural schedule. Her days routinely were thirty-six to thirty-eight hours long, and her nights, ten to twelve hours. She felt so good on this schedule that she abandoned her attempts to be a 9:00-to-5:00 journalist and became a freelance writer instead.

Not all insomnias are simple one-cause problems with a single magic solution. Quitting a sleeping pill, for example, can be complicated business. On the one hand, there is the medical problem of withdrawing the drug from the body, and on the other hand, there is the behavioral habit of taking the pill as part of your bedtime routine. And there are other problems difficult to solve because they are impossible to explain.

The pseudoinsomnias fall into this category. These are genuine mysteries to the sleep expert because a patient may be complaining of a serious sleep problem but, as far as all the sleep recordings show, he or she is getting a perfectly normal night's sleep. There was a time when the sleep-watchers chose to believe what their machines recorded, not what the patient said. People who claimed they hardly slept, when the polygraph said they did, were either hypochondriacs or, like the character Captain Flume in Joseph Heller's *Catch-22*, were just dreaming they were awake—at least that's what the sleep doctors thought.

Now the experts are taking these complaints much more seriously because, for one thing, they're beginning to find they've been missing a few symptoms in some of their patients. It turns out that some people do have naturally feeble sleep. Or, as was mentioned in the first chapter, the minds of others are still alert during sleep, or suffering from alpha-wave pollution while they sleep.

Because many of these pseudoinsomnias are genuine, the sleep clinicians are also beginning to realize the limits of their measuring equipment. There are nuances to a night's sleep that are still too subtle for the sleep machines to pick up in the problem cases. What is a barely detectable scribble on the sleep recording might stand for a sleep defect that is keeping your mind awake for most of the night. The sleep doctors now realize how elusive these insomnias can be, so they take a long, hard look at all problems, even the ones that don't show up on their equipment. "When my machine says a person slept, and he says he didn't, it's not grounds for saying he's wrong," says Dr. Hauri. "Now we are finding all kinds of things wrong with these pseudoinsomniacs who were supposed to have nothing wrong with them except being complainers."

Many pseudoinsomniacs have now graduated to another group, the idiopathic insomniacs who are known to have a real insomnia, but for reasons no one has deciphered as yet. In this group belong the people whose sleep is a series of miniawakenings or interruptions, who have trouble with alpha waves in their sleep, who are naturally tense sleepers, or who sleep in a state of hyperalert thinking.

These problem cases are making the sleep-watchers take a closer look at how you sleep. What they're finding out is that sleep is much more complicated than they thought. "A person can be both awake and asleep," says Montefiore's Dr. Pollok. "They're not mutually exclusive states. The brain is a tremendously complex organ; different parts of it can be in different states at various times. If everything in it is well coordinated, you can say that you're awake, or you're asleep. But even then, there are transitional periods, dreamy periods in the morning, for example, when you're in a borderland between sleeping and waking."

"In people who have defective sleep," he continues, "that kind of organization is disturbed. When that happens, you see twilight behavior, twilight feelings. We already know that people who are narcoleptics can be constantly in this twilight world, with part of them awake, part of them asleep."

It's the twilight people who are providing some of the challenge to the sleep clinics and stimulating more research into sleep problems in general and insomnia in particular. At the Dartmouth sleep clinic, for example, Dr. Hauri now has two kinds of biofeedback that help some of the idiopathic insomniacs into a peaceful night's sleep. For those that seem too tense, too aroused to rest, he uses a biofeedback machine that monitors a person's muscle tension and, by a series of clicking signals, tells him or her when the body is too taut. The higher the muscle tension, the more clicks from the machine. With a little practice, the insomniacs learn to uncoil and relax themselves, making sleep come a little more easily.

For people who just seem to have naturally rotten sleep, Dr. Hauri has another biofeedback system that uses a delicate, ultrasensitive machine that monitors a specific kind of brain wave which appears in stage-2 sleep. It is a brief, intense spurt of electric activity called a sleep spindle. People with miserable sleep seem to have few of these while they rest. By watching the brain-wave machine, poor sleepers learn when they are producing these special sleep spindles and, after a little practice, they figure out how to manipulate those inner controls that will give them more of these waves and more sleep. Dr. Hauri has good luck with his biofeedback methods if he connects the right kind of insomniac to the right machine. In one test with eighteen people, all of whom had insomnia for at least two years, he connected the tense sleepers to his muscle tension machine and the naturally bad sleepers to his SMR (for sensorimotor) machine, which measures sleep spindles. By using his special biofeedback equipment, he was able to not only help them sleep longer and more soundly, but also to reduce by almost half the average amount of time it took them to get to sleep.

Before you run out and spend money on a biofeedback gadget, you should know that, first of all, the SMR machine is not available. It is a highly sophisticated piece of equipment that was especially designed for this type of research and not for the open market. Secondly, most biofeedback devices you can buy measure alpha waves, the kind your brain makes when you're relaxed but awake. So far, researchers have found that these types do nothing to help you sleep. Once you hit the alpha state, you may be relaxed, but you're still apt not to sleep if you have insomnia. Lastly, many of these machines are not of the highest quality, even the ones in the $100-plus price range. A writer friend of mine who was doing a story on biofeedback found this out with the help of his small daughter and a grapefruit.

A machine manufacturer had loaned him what it said was one of its top-notch biofeedback devices to help with his research. My friend brought the gadget home, where his wife, who did yoga every day, tried it out. She settled into one of her relaxing poses and put on the headband attached to the machine. Instantly she was pumping out alpha waves—the machine told her so with its gentle "Boop-Boop-Boop" sound. My friend tried on the headband and in seconds he heard the same sound, "Boop-Boop-Boop." Then his two-year-old daughter walked into the room, carrying a grapefruit. My friend put the headband on the grapefruit—"Boop-Boop-Boop."

"Either I had a very serene grapefruit," he said later, "or I had a bum machine." The moral of the story is that if they offer you biofeedback in the sleep clinic, take it. But if you plan to get one for home use, be prepared to be disappointed.

At Montefiore Hospital's sleep clinic they are also trying out new therapies, some applicable to victims of sleep apnea. Having the patient sleep upright in an easy chair instead of a bed, for example, seems to help some people, while others' breathing problems seem to clear up if they go on a diet. (Overweight men tend to be more apnea-prone.)

To find out what makes your body clock tick, Montefiore scientists are studying how it functions naturally in a timeless world. Volunteers have lived in windowless rooms for three and a half weeks while in the next room machines connected to them monitor their brain waves, body temperature shifts, and sleep habits on a minute-by-minute basis, twenty-four hours a day. The laboratory even has a kind of mechanical vampire connected to a vein in the people's arms. Every now and then it takes a sip of blood to study hormone content and do various tests on it. Short of climbing inside a person's skin, this is probably the closest that science will get to observing the complicated rhythms of the body in action.

What has been discovered is that, left to itself, the body does seem to have its own twenty-five-hour day and some of its "days" can stretch out to as long as thirty-six hours, as in the case of Dr. Hauri's female journalist, with "nights" that last as long as sixteen hours of sleep. In spite of this, some rhythms, such as those involving temperature shifts, mental alertness, and abilities to concentrate, seem to remain faithful to a twenty-four-hour day even when the person is shut off from the cues of night and day. Somewhere in the mountain of information these tests are producing, the researchers expect to find the answers to basic questions about an individual's sleep personality, such as what makes one sleeper a lark and another an owl.

Keeping someone locked in a room for three and a half weeks is an interesting way to study body rhythms but not a very practical way to diagnose any problems with them. One of the big difficulties with watching body rhythms is that the best way to study them has not been the most convenient way. The most accurate measure of your tempo shifts is your rectal temperature, and the best way to check it is every few minutes around the clock. Charting these changes gives a clear picture of when your body has its "days"—temperature highs— and "nights"—temperature lows.

The Montefiore experts were faced with this problem when they had one insomniac patient with a body clock that just wouldn't conform to the normal day. He was running on his own twenty-five-hour day and had been for the past eight years. It ruined his chances for normal living and even work. He had been unable to hold down a job for the two years prior to his admission to the Montefiore program.

To get a more detailed picture of his body rhythms, the sleep clinicians decided to use a robot. For three and a half months the man wore a small rectal thermometer attached to a small computer he carried around in his pocket. Every six minutes of every day the computer took his temperature and memorized it. About twice a week the man would report to the clinic where his small electronic brain would transmit all the temperature information to a master computer which was keeping a running record of all the temperature shifts.

At the end of the months the records showed that the man was sleeping normal amounts of sleep but at very strange times. Bedtime could be anywhere from noon to eight at night. It was a tremendously erratic day and one that would have never been uncovered without the help of the little robot. (Montefiore scientists have since used it to keep total all-day records of other specific functions, such as changes in a person's heartbeat and changes in a woman's body around ovulation time.)

The most interesting part of the man's case wasn't the robot watching him, or the fact that he felt like going to sleep when everyone else was having lunch. It was the cure.

The sleep experts had their thousands of computer-recorded temperature readings. They had carefully mapped out charts of the man's shifting days and nights. They had a meticulous day-by-day diary of his activities that they had all studied closely. They took all this raw data, pored over it, discussed it with each other, and gradually pieced together a plan of action to try to put the man's body in step with the normal day.

Just as they were ready to start treatment, the man suddenly but smoothly shifted over to a twenty-four-hour day, all by himself. When I asked one of the doctors involved in the case why, after eight years, the man's body suddenly cured itself, he replied, "Well, we've got a lot of theories about what happened here, but, practically speaking, we really don't know." Which indicates that, as good as sleep clinics are and as far as we've come in understanding sleep, we still have a few things left to learn.

4.
The Search
for the Perfect Pill

As long as there has been insomnia, there has always been *the* foolproof cure. For the ancient Greeks and Romans, it was spending a night in the temple of their favorite god. That was replaced by magic sleep potions made of every thing from mandrake to lettuce juice. Probably the most spectacular and grisly of guaranteed sleep inducers was something called the Hand of Glory, very big in medieval Europe. It was a candle holder made from the mummified hand of a man who had been hanged. It was designed to hold a special kind of candle, one made from the fat of another criminal who also had been hanged. The black magic theory behind using all these recycled parts was that anyone who stared at the candle's flickering flame was supposed to sink into a deep stupor. This was the medieval equivalent of Seconal.

Of course now we are much more sophisticated. We don't look at our sleep inducers, we swallow them. And we swallow them by the millions. According to one government survey, drugstores filled over 27 million prescriptions for sleeping pills alone in 1976. At an average of forty pills per bottle, that is a little over a billion doses, enough to knock out everyone in the United States for four nights. How many of the nonprescription drugs, or OTC (for over-the-counter) sleeping pills like Sominex and Nytol were also purchased that same year is not known, but according to Dr. Milton Kramer, Professor of Psychiatry at the University of Cincinnati College of Medicine, insomniacs have enough faith in any and all sleeping pills to generate about $175 million of annual income for the sleeping pill industry. Before you contribute your few dollars to this booming business, you might want to know a little bit about what you're buying.

It has only been in the past ten years or so that sleep experts have been taking a close look at just how good sleeping pills are. And what they've found is that there is much less than meets the eye in just about every pill available these days. For one thing, it looks as though we have been giving the pills too much credit for working when they did, and not enough credit to ourselves.

As a nation of sufferers, we have what amounts to a religious belief in the power of the pill. We take tablets and capsules for everything from anxiety, backaches, colds, depression, fatigue, hangovers, heartburn, and stomachaches to, of course, insomnia. If one pill doesn't work, we don't lose faith. We just change pills. The power of this belief is awesome and still very mysterious. How effective a drug is depends only partially on its chemical content. The drug has to appeal to you. You have to believe in it, which is one reason why some of the deadliest medication may be packaged in cheery gelatin shells of candy-bright reds, yellows, and greens, and why you don't see many gray or black pills.

This belief is called the placebo (meaning I will be pleasing in Latin) effect, and it can turn any dud, fake sugar pill into a wonder drug just by your faith in it. It's so real and so powerful that drug companies routinely match-test new drugs against placebos, or sugar pills, to make sure the drugs work well enough on their own. Just the act of taking a pill has a special, powerful effect.

Two Yale psychologists, Michael Storm and William Nisbett, did an ingenious experiment showing this placebo power in action with a group of insomniacs. The people were told that they were part of a dream research group and that in the course of study they would be given a safe, nonprescription drug that would in no way interfere with their daily work. It was in fact a fake placebo pill with all the chemical potency of a glass of water.

The group was told that the pill they were getting was a mild stimulant they would take before bedtime. It would start their minds racing, quicken their pulse, and send adrenalin surging into their system—symptoms identical to those the insomniacs had complained about in a preexperiment interview. All of the insomniacs were caught up in a vicious cycle of staying awake and being restless because they were worried. And they were worried because they had been awake and restless.

After taking what they thought was some kind of stimulant, the insomniacs fell asleep twelve minutes *sooner* than usual. The reason for this, said Storm and Nisbett, was something they tagged "reverse attribution." The insomniacs believed it was the pill, not their worrying, that kept them awake. As a result, they were more relaxed and went to sleep more quickly.

Of course the placebo effect works the way you would expect it to as well, giving pills knockout power long after they've become impotent. According to psychologist Dr. Stephen Spielman of Montefiore Hospital in New York, the most common kind of drug abuse that eventually brings the insomniac to the sleep clinic for a cure is pill-swapping, skipping from one drug to another in search of a night's sleep. Eventually, insomniacs use these drugs so often that they become immune to their chemical effects. The odd thing is that even though the drugs aren't supposed to work and put the user to sleep, they often do, especially if the insomniac had just made a pill change. Popping a different kind of pill, says Spielman, actually changes the users' attitude toward their sleep and temporarily distracts them from the worry and agitation that have been keeping them awake. When one of these people shows up at a sleep clinic, the experts are faced with the problem of weaning him or her off a sleep drug which can sometimes be physically addicting, and they have to break the hold of this placebo effect, which has a kind of psychological addiction all its own.

For these reasons, and others which will be described in grim detail later in this chapter, try *anything* within reason before you turn to a sleeping pill or any kind of drug, including alcohol. Especially alcohol. In most cases you stand to lose more than you will gain, and you can generate your own placebo effect without any pill. There's really not much to be said in favor of sleeping pills, but if you are determined to use them, or already have some, take the time to read through the rest of this chapter.

Your choices are from two categories: the OTC (Over-the-counter) nonprescription pills you buy off the shelf in your drugstore; and the prescription pills that your doctor recommends to you. Most novice pill-takers start with the OTC, nonprescription drugs because they seem so safe and because of all those serene, smiling TV actors who confide to you that they sometimes have trouble sleeping and get help from that bottle of pills that's flashed on the screen. The kindest thing that can be said about these types of sleep aids is that they won't kill you. In addition to that, they're a waste of money. You stand a better chance of getting to sleep by taking the money you were going to spend on these pills and getting a dull paperback for bedtime reading instead.

The big problem with all the OTC sleeping pills is that, in recommended doses, they don't work. In one test run at Pennsylvania State University, sleep expert Dr. Anthony Kales matched the recommended doses of a leading OTC sleeping pill against a placebo in ten insomniacs. The OTC pill didn't do any better than the sugar pill in getting the insomniacs to sleep or improving their sleep. In the words of the study, "the drug produced no favorable effects."

The second problem is that to get any serious help getting to sleep you have to take more of the drugs than the manufacturer specifies, a move that would expose you to dangerous side effects from the drugs used in these pills. The main ingredients in most OTC sleeping pills are either a substance called scopolamine, or antihistamines which are variously labeled as methapyrilene hydrochloride or methapyrilene fumarate.

Scopolamine is the chief ingredient in common OTC pills. Taking more than the standard dose may not only do little to help you sleep, it will also intensify the side effects of taking a normal dose. Blurred vision, dry mouth, difficulty in urination, and pressure in the eyes (potentially dangerous if you have glaucoma and don't know it) are possible side effects of a recommended dose. Confusion, excitement, and even delirium can come with heavier doses.

Other OTC sleeping pills all have antihistamines as their main ingredients. Sometimes the pills are laced with a little scopolamine for added effect; in other instances, the antihistamines are thrown in as an added ingredient.

As you probably already know, antihistamines are also the prime ingredients in many of those cold capsules with all their tiny pills. You also may recall that the label warnings on these cold remedies caution users not to drink any alcohol with the pills and not to operate any machinery because the pills may cause a side effect of drowsiness. The drug companies have repackaged this side effect and turned it into a whole new product, the nonprescription sleeping pill. The antihistamine OTC pill may help you sleep if your insomnia is caused by an allergy problem such as hay fever. (The prime medical use of these drugs is in treating allergies.) But if that's not your problem, you'll be getting basically the same sleep-inducing effect of the scopolamine drugs, which is practically nil.

In either case, what you get when you buy an OTC sleeping pill is something truly unique, a product with all the benefits of a placebo, or sugar pill, and with the risks of a real drug. The general feeling among many doctors, especially sleep experts, is that these drugs are, practically speaking, useless and potentially dangerous. In testimony before a Senate subcommittee investigating the wisdom of leaving the OTC pills out in the nonprescription market, sleeping pill expert Dr. David Greenblatt of Massachusetts General Hospital in Boston claimed that, at best, the pills were only mild sedatives.

In high doses they were potentially dangerous, since they could trigger hallucinations and delirium, as well as raise the body's temperature and blood pressure to dangerous levels. And in his testimony before the committee, Dr. Anthony Kales went as far as recommending that the pills be pulled off the market because they were potentially dangerous and were so heavily oversold. The basic message of the pill commercials, he said, was that no one should tolerate even an occasional problem with sleeping, but should instead try to obliterate it with one of these pills.

A Food and Drug Administration panel of experts essentially agreed, and although it didn't suggest taking the pills off the shelves, it did recommend that every package of pills carry the following warnings:

• Do not take any OTC drug along with a prescription drug without the advice of a doctor or pharmacist. Antihistamines, for example, enhance the stupefying effects of tranquilizers and sedatives, as well as other medications containing antihistamines.

• Do not give them to children under twelve.
• Take them with caution if you drink. (Alcohol may put you in a deeper stupor.)
• Consult a doctor if the insomnia persists for more than two weeks.

What would be even better would be a fifth warning:

• You can save yourself the trouble of having to remember all of the warnings above by not even bothering with the pills.

But if your insomnia is getting to you so much that you're ready to go out and get a pill for it, maybe you should save your money and go to a doctor for the high-potency type, the prescription pill. Unlike the OTC pills, prescription drugs are practically guaranteed to work, for a short while. They are also guaranteed to expose you to plenty of dangers if you use them carelessly, so it is not a decision you should make lightly.

Whether you take the pills is really up to you. Although they are only supposed to be doled out by prescription, getting them usually requires nothing more than showing up at the doctor's office to be handed that slip of paper. "If you've got the right complaint," says one antipill sleep clinician, "practically any doctor will give them to you. The pills are easy to get." And you'll probably get them pretty quickly as well. According to Dr. William Dement of the Stanford University Sleep Clinic, the average amount of time a doctor spends on an insomnia complaint is about three minutes. In defense of the doctors, one reason for this fast-food approach to handing out prescriptions is the number of insomniacs they see. One estimate is that close to one-fifth of all office visits are made by people seeking sleeping pills.

As was mentioned in an earlier chapter, you should seek out some kind of professional help to deal with your insomnia if it has developed to the point where it interferes seriously with how you function during the day, and has been a nightly problem for two weeks or more. You may very well know what is causing your insomnia. If you do, make sure to tell your doctor. He or she might be able to help you get a decent night's sleep without resorting to a sleeping pill.

Sometimes just a mild dose of sedatives taken during the day or a nightly dose of an antidepressant will be all that is necessary to get you a good night's sleep. If these don't seem appropriate to your problem, your doctor may turn to the sleeping pill or, as it is called in medical jargon, the hypnotic.

Your doctor has over sixty different sleep drugs to choose from, but whatever he or she picks, it will fall into one of three general drug categories: the barbiturates; a grab-bag group called nonbarbiturates; and the benzodiazepines. (For help in picking your way through the muddle of names, you will find a chart of the most commonly prescribed pills on page 175.) Like the characters in a Russian novel, every hypnotic has at least two names: an official generic name that describes the predominant drug used in the pill, and the trade name (or brand name) put on the pill by the manufacturer. The total number of names varies from one pill to another. The sleeping pill known under the generic name of phenobarbital, for example, travels under about a dozen different trade names as well.

In the past ten years or so sleep experts have been testing some of the more common prescription drugs and have found that the various drugs are not as different as they might seem. As it turns out, sleeping pills have many features in common. Four important ones that you should know about before taking any kind of prescription sleep aid are:

• No pill gives you a completely normal night's sleep. All prescription pills are CNS (for Central Nervous System) depressants, which is a technical way of saying that they work by going straight to your brain and knocking you unconscious. They lower your heart rate, blood pressure, rate of breathing, reflexes, and muscle tone. They also wipe out part of your sleep, usually the REM cycles.

• All sleeping pills are only temporary solutions to insomnia. Every pill will put you out the first few evenings, but, taken nightly, most lose their power in two weeks or less.

• When you quit taking any sleeping pill, you have to go through drug withdrawal. This is true if you take a pill for one night or ten nights. One of the common withdrawal effects is insomnia, and, depending on the size of the dose and how long you were taking the pill, the effects could linger for a few days or for months.

• Any sleeping pill will *cause* insomnia if you take it long enough. A sleeping pill habit carried on too long can totally disrupt your natural sleep process to the point where your insomnia will be worse than it was before you began taking the pill.

Many of these discoveries were made simply by studying people who got in the habit of taking pills for months, even years, to cure their insomnias and who suffered the consequences. The reports of sleep clinics are full of examples of those who found these features of pills out the hard way.

One of the more spectacular cases was the fifty-eight-year-old man who was about to self-destruct from a heavy sleeping pill–alcohol habit. It started when he got a big job promotion as a young man and he began losing sleep over the problems and worries that came with it. To help him get to sleep, he got a barbiturate sleeping pill prescription from his doctor and began taking it steadily. That was back in 1941.

By the time he came to the sleep clinic thirty years later, he was taking three kinds of pills—two sleeping pills and one sedative—every night in triple and quadruple doses as part of his bedtime routine. On nights when those didn't work, he swallowed whole handfuls of pills and washed them down with close to a fifth of whiskey. As a result, he had total blackouts and passed out from the overdose. During at least four of these blackouts his wife had to drag him to the hospital to bring him back to consciousness. Once he spent five days in a coma before coming around.

It was after the last blackout that he decided to get help from the sleep clinic. A night in the laboratory showed he didn't really sleep as much as sink into a stupor. Brain-wave recordings showed that he had no normal sleep during any part of the night. He had to be sent to the hospital to free him of what was now an addiction to sleeping pills. Alcoholics Anonymous helped get him off drinking whiskey to go to sleep, and the man had to go into therapy to learn how to rebuild ties with family and friends that had been destroyed by his drug habits. He took biofeedback training to help relax and was prescribed some mild antidepressants to help him cope. This whole process took about six months and for the first time in thirty years gave him about five hours of normal sleep at night.

You probably think the story of this man was included here to scare you a little. And you're right. Sleeping pills are highly potent drugs. You can never be too careful about how you use them. This man's case is not typical of many who have overused pills because his abuse was on such a spectacular scale. What is typical is that he was not only trying many different pills and drugs but also relied on a very common nonsleep drug, alcohol. What is also typical is that he was taking enough to kill the average person, and almost did kill himself.

What saved him was something called tolerance, a medical term meaning that his body developed immunity to both the lethal and sleep-inducing effects of the drugs. Doctors have been aware of this phenomenon since at least the 1930s, when barbiturate sleeping pills were commonly used. They knew that, after a while, the effectiveness of a dose of sleeping pills would fade and they would have to increase the amount of drugs to get the same effect.

It wasn't until 1970 that anyone actually took the time to find out exactly how long each of the sleeping pills worked before the human body developed tolerance to it. That year, psychiatrist Dr. Anthony Kales of Penn State University published the results of a study he did with pills from each of the main drug groups—the barbiturates, non-barbiturates, and benzodiazepines. Every night for fourteen nights he watched the sleep of a group of insomniacs who volunteered to take a normal dose of the sleep drugs at bedtime. None of them had taken any pills or even alcohol before the experiment, so everyone started on equal footing. What Kales found was that by the end of the two weeks all the drugs but one, a benzodiazepine pill called Dalmane, had lost most or all of their sleep-inducing powers. One drug, a non-barbiturate named chloral hydrate, stopped working after only three days. Further tests have shown that the one drug that made it to the end of the two weeks, Dalmane, keeps working at the same dosage for about five or six weeks.

In spite of these discoveries, many doctors today are still giving their insomniac patients more sleeping pills than are good for them. According to a survey done by the National Institute on Drug Abuse, in 1976 the average prescription for barbiturate sleeping pills was for a thirty- to forty-day supply. This means that even if you follow your doctor's orders, you might be taking pills long after they've stopped doing you any good.

When they're working, all the pills will affect the way you sleep. Barbiturate and nonbarbiturate sleeping pills jam your natural sleep mechanism so that you have no REM cycles when you rest at night. A single sleeping pill can wipe out REM dream periods for as long as one or two nights after you've taken it. This doesn't create a problem while you're on the pill, but once you've quit, your brain goes through a withdrawal process in which all those blocked-up REM cycles come rushing back. On the nights after you've gone off a pill, your brain has an orgy of dreams and even nightmares, and your sleep is shallow and not very restful.

If you've taken the pill for a short amount of time, this is usually just a minor inconvenience. If you've been taking pills frequently (for instance, every night for two weeks or more) and then quit, this onrush of REM sleep, called REM rebound, can be so disturbing (especially if it brings a lot of nightmares) that it can cause insomnia and even drive you back to the pill. What is even stranger is that you may have these withdrawal effects while you are still taking a sleeping pill. What has happened is that your body has developed a tolerance to your present dose and the process of the REM rebound starts with a nightly glut of dreaming and nightmares.

According to Dr. Kales, it often happens that some pill-taking insomniacs don't realize that the nightmares they have are part of a natural biochemical reaction of withdrawal. Instead, they mistake them for being symptoms of some deep psychological disturbances struggling to get out. To escape these nightly horrors, some people boost their intake of pills, sometimes to an overdose level.

The REM rebound of sleeping pill withdrawal can expose you to other risks as well. Asthma victims may suffer increased nightly asthma attacks triggered by extra REM sleep cycles. Since REM sleep also brings with it a surge of gastric acid, ulcer victims may have their sleep interrupted by painful ulcer attacks during REM sleep. People with heart conditions face a special risk, because one of the physical side effects of REM sleep is a faster heartbeat. The overload of intense heart work that comes with a REM rebound could be too much for a weak heart.

Dr. Anthony Kales had one patient who had thirty-two angina attacks during just one withdrawal night. For this reason, University of Oklahoma sleep researcher Dr. William Orr says that doctors should be especially careful about prescribing sleeping pills to their heart patients and withdrawing them.

People with nighttime breathing problems are also high-risk candidates during sleeping pill use, mainly because the depression of breathing is one of the drugs' routine side effects. If your insomnia is caused by sleep apnea in which your breath stops completely throughout the night or if it's caused by suffocating asthma attacks, the last thing you need is a drug that interferes with what few breaths you do get.

Withdrawal effects will cause insomnia for a few days after you've quit a sleeping pill, even if you've only used it for a short time. The same effects can linger for weeks or even months if you are a heavy pill-user. What is worse, you can destroy what little sleep you get while you're taking the very pills that are supposed to help you sleep. At his sleep laboratory Dr. Kales did a comparison study of two groups of insomniacs, each carefully matched by age and background. Each had complained of suffering from insomnia for about the same number of years, but the big difference between them was that one group had been taking sleeping pills for their problem, while the other hadn't.

After studying their sleep for a few nights, Dr. Kales found that those who had been taking pills slept worse than the pill-free insomniacs. The pill-takers took longer to get to sleep, woke more frequently during the night, and had less REM sleep. All they had accomplished by taking the pills for so long (in some instances, as long as ten years) was to make worse a problem they were trying to eliminate. As they went to bed every night they were actually swallowing the cause of their insomnia.

Developing a heavy sleeping pill habit exposes you to another very common risk, dependency. All the barbiturates, and some of the non-barbiturates as well, can be physically addicting. Insomniacs may come to need their sleep drugs the way alcoholics need their drink or junkies need their needle. When this happens, you can't quit the pill without taking serious medical risks. Less dangerous, but still a big problem with long-term pill use, is psychological dependency on the drug. Even though it no longer works for you and may even be ruining your sleep, the pill becomes a necessary part of your bedtime ritual. You become convinced that if you take away the pill you will sleep even worse than you do now. Sleep clinicians have found that they have to wean pill-takers off this psychological dependency as well the physical addiction of the sleep drug in order to cure heavy habits.

However long or short a time you use a sleeping pill, another effect you'll always have to cope with is the hangover effect the morning after a pill night. There's a lingering stupor when you get up in the morning that may cling to you for part of the day. It can hang on for as long as eighteen hours after you've taken the drug. This means that if you take a pill at 11:00 at night before bedtime, you could still be a little hazy from the drug as late as 5:00 P.M. the following day.

Although people do mix and match, prescription pills are too potent to combine with other similar drugs—sleeping pills, sedatives, tranquilizers, or alcohol. The reason is something called the synergistic effect, in which the total effect of two or more drugs is greater than the sum of the combination's parts. It's sometimes called the "1 + 1 = 3" effect. That's one reason why using a little alcohol to wash down a sleeping pill can be a dangerous, almost suicidal, habit. What you end up with is a more stupefying, but still not very satisfying, sleep. You also must face a bigger hangover the next morning, and a bigger risk of overdosing.

One last complication that comes with taking pills applies to anyone over sixty. For some reason, older people react more strongly to minimal standard doses of hypnotics, sometimes in perverse or strange ways. Some become too sleepy and too depressed with a standard dose, while others may become agitated, confused, even a little delerious. The reason for this isn't clear, but one theory is that older peoples' systems don't absorb and break down the drugs as quickly and efficiently as do those of younger people. Whatever the reason, drug companies routinely advise doctors to use the smallest dose on insomniacs over sixty until it is clear how they react.

There was a time when the only pills doctors would prescribe to their patients were one kind or another of barbiturates. Barbiturates were considered wonder drugs in their time, around the turn of the century. According to Consumers Union, in 1903 two German chemists, von Mering and Fischer, marketed a sedative–sleeping pill named Veronal that was made from the synthetic chemical barbital. The barbiturates were born. They revolutionized the sleeping pill business, which at that time was practically nonexistent. The two most common cures for insomnia in the early 1900s were alcohol and the drug chloral hydrate, which some found objectionable because it had a bitter taste and upset their stomachs.

For those who didn't like the taste of chloral hydrate or who didn't drink, the barbiturates seemed like the ideal solution. Not only were they odorless and tasteless, but, unlike alcohol, they could be given in precise dosages with no fuss, no muss. They proved to be such a success that over the years more than 2,500 barbiturate drugs were synthesized. It looked like the ideal sleeping pill had been discovered.

The optimism didn't last, however, because the barbiturates proved to be vicious, unforgiving drugs to those who abused them. According to a 1977 report by the National Institute on Drug Abuse on the use and abuse of sleeping pills and sedatives, about 5,000 people die each year from barbiturate overdoses or with barbiturates as a contributing cause. The institute also found that close to one-fifth of all drug deaths in 1976 involved sleeping pills, with barbiturates accounting for the lion's share. What was stunning about the figure was that it very nearly equalled the percentage of deaths from heroin for the same year. In addition to all these fatalities, misuse of barbiturates was also responsible for sending about 25,000 people to hospital emergency rooms that same year. The wonder drug had become a real killer.

The reason barbiturates have proved to be so dangerous is because they are addictive drugs. It only takes a few weeks of steady use to develop a physical dependency, and once you do, you need a doctor's help to withdraw. Heavy barbiturate users should never try quitting on their own. Going cold turkey can be extremely dangerous, because withdrawal from barbiturates is even more difficult and dangerous than heroin withdrawal.

Routine withdrawal symptoms include daytime jitters, the "shakes," anxiety, and nervousness. In more extreme cases, there may also be hallucinations, convulsions, delirium, fevers, and hypertension. In some instances the doctor has to give the barbiturate-user another kind of sleeping pill to help him or her make it through the dream- and nightmare-filled nights. The process of withdrawal can be long and arduous. Dr. William Dement of Stanford University reported the case of one woman who had been taking six different kinds of sleep drugs for over thirty years. It took a total of two years to withdraw her from all of them.

Barbiturates are also dangerous because the difference between a normal dose and a lethal dose is not all that great. Drug specialists call this difference the margin of safety, and with barbiturates it is a relatively thin line. The hazards of this are that a person does not have to take much more than the standard dose to be exposed to the dangers of a lethal overdose. This is a fact known to many would-be suicides, since secobarbital, one of the barbiturates, is one of the most popular suicide drugs, according the National Institute of Drug Abuse (NIDA). Taking other sleeping pills, sedatives, or alcohol narrows this margin even more because of the "1 + 1 = 3" effect. In general, the Institute concludes that those who use barbiturates, even for legitimate medical purposes, face a higher than average risk of accidental death.

One last complication that comes with barbiturates stems from the way they interact and sometimes interfere with other drugs. They may suppress some of the pain-killing effects of aspirin, for example, so that you may have to take larger doses to get rid of a headache. They also change the body's metabolism so that other drugs—such as birth control pills, cortisone, and anticoagulants that stroke victims may take to clear clots from their system—are discarded from the body much more quickly than they should be. Your doctor should be aware of all these complications, but if you have any doubt about taking a barbiturate with any other medication, be sure to ask.

Because there are drug alternatives now, many doctors have stopped prescribing barbiturates for their insomniac patients. Most probably agree with Drs. Jan Koch-Weser and David Greenblatt, who wrote in the *New England Journal of Medicine:* "The barbiturate hypnotics have been rendered obsolete by pharmacologic progress and deserve speedy oblivion." Because of this attitude change, the chances are better than average that whatever sleeping pill your doctor gives you won't be a barbiturate, so you won't have to worry about the problems and risks that come with it.

What you may get is something out of the second group of sleeping pills, called the nonbarbiturates. These began appearing in the mid-1950s, when it started to become obvious that the barbiturates were not the wonder drugs everyone thought they were. The most commonly used are the drugs ethchlorvynol, glutethimide, methaqualone, and methyprylon. Also included in this group is the old nineteenth-century drug chloral hydrate, still used by many doctors.

These nonbarbiturates were originally designed to replace the dangerous barbiturates, but it turned out that they were more of the same kind of pill. Not only did they have the same burn-out rate as barbiturates, the same REM sleep-blocking effects, the same withdrawal problems and hangovers, and the same effects on those over sixty, they also had many of the same medical dangers as well. All but chloral hydrate have a small margin of error in their dose levels; they are dangerous when taken with alcohol; they can be as addictive as the barbiturates; and they can interfere with the working of other drugs. The nonbarbiturates also present a few problems of their own.

Chloral hydrate is not as dangerous as the other nonbarbiturates in combination with alcohol, but taken over a long stretch of time it can cause kidney damage, physical dependence, and ulcers. Ethchlorvynol not only interferes with anticoagulants, but it can also trigger delerium when taken with antidepressant drugs sometimes prescribed to insomniacs. Glutethimide, according to the National Institute on Drug Abuse, was an even higher risk drug than many of the barbiturates. On a one-to-ten rating of the most dangerous sleeping pills, it was number three. Finally, methaqualone, probably best known under the trade name Quaalude, has become such a heavily abused drug among the young that many drug stores now refuse to carry it rather than contribute to the abuse. In some ways these drugs are even more dangerous than the barbiturates, because doctors have less experience working with their side effects and, more importantly, have less experience in treating overdose victims. Except for chloral hydrate, all nonbarbiturates are basically the same old barbiturates with some new problems added. A panel of experts asked by the NIDA to study and evaluate the nonbarbiturate drugs concluded, on the basis of the facts, that "there was little justification for the continued use of these compounds."

One reason for this opinion was the development of a third group of drugs called the benzodiazepines, which includes the tranquilizers Valium and Librium and a relatively new sleeping pill, flurazepam, known under the trade name Dalmane. Dalmane is an improvement over all the other pills and is probably your best bet right now among prescription sleep drugs. Among Dalmane's advantages are that it doesn't bother your REM sleep at all; it doesn't slow down your breathing; it doesn't interfere with other drugs; and it works longer than the other pills—about three to four weeks longer. Doctors report that patients have less trouble withdrawing from the pill and it is generally not as dangerous as the other drugs. People have taken as much as eleven times the normal dose and survived. In tests with animals, scientists weren't even able to determine what the lethal dose of Dalmane might be. According to two doctors, the only way researchers could kill a lab animal with the drug was "to smother it with a mound of tablets."

This is still not the perfect pill. Dalmane wipes out the deep, restful, stage-4 sleep. It also has a strong hangover effect, cannot be taken with alcohol, and can trigger odd reactions in people over sixty. Although it is not physically addictive, as the barbiturates are, like all sleeping pills it can cause a psychological dependence which is almost as strong as physical addiction. Finally, it is a relatively young drug— less than ten years old—and for that reason doctors are cautious about hailing it as the sleeping pill of the future. It is still possible there is some devastating side effect to the pill that has not yet been discovered. But for the moment it is ahead of the others.

"Dalmane, by all standards, is the 'best' pill," says Dr. Charles Pollok of New York's Montefiore Hospital. "It's the one that's both the most effective and that has the longest lasting effects; but we aren't talking about long-term treatment, say a year long. It only lasts for about five or six weeks." What it really comes down to is that, after more than seventy years of making sleeping pills, drug researchers have come up with a not-too-dangerous sleeping pill that works for about a month and a half.

This is the sleeping pill situation as it exists today. If you approach it with a realistic sense of what you can get from the average sleep drug, you will be able to enjoy a reasonably satisfactory night's rest without any serious troubles. As long as you are aware that you can't cure insomnia with a pill, and that every pill gives you a partial sleep and brings a few side effects with it, and as long as you follow the dose schedule that comes with the prescription, you should have nothing to worry about.

Are sleeping pills worth using at all? It depends on whom you ask. The NIDA report on sleeping pills says they have some value for relieving an insomniac's sleep problems over a short (six weeks or less) period of time. The head of a large metropolitan sleep clinic was asked the same question one night on a TV health show about in-somnia. His answer? "In certain special circumstances, where there is a need for short-term management, sleeping pills can be useful. How-ever in long term, chronic insomnia, it's not been demonstrated that they work. In fact there are now cases in which it's been shown that it can actually cause chronic insomnia."

A few days later I was talking to one of his colleagues. The pill question came up. "Sleeping pills?" he answered. "Well, the current line goes something like this: 'Long-term, high-dose sleeping pills have been shown to be harmful and even counterproductive. They've even been shown to be causes of insomnia. Furthermore, long-term use of sleeping pills has never been shown to be effective; but certain sleep-ing pills have been shown to be effective in the short run. Perhaps this is the area where they have some use.'" He said it in almost a single breath, like a child reciting a well-memorized lesson. "'The truth is," he continued, "we don't know that there's *any* place for sleeping pills. We just don't know that for sure."

A couple of arguments against using pills to fight insomnia are offered by Dr. Thomas Roth and his fellow sleep clinicians at the University of Cincinnati. The first is that sleeping pills may only really treat half of an insomnia. There are two basic measures of sleep: the objective kind that the sleep lab makes with its machines; and the subjective kind, basically a matter of how well you *think* you slept the next morning. They can be two entirely different sleeps.

As evidence, Dr. Roth and his colleagues offer a comparison study they did in which they watched one group of normal sleepers and one group of insomniacs rest for a few nights. On the following morn-ings, most of the good sleepers were able to estimate within ten or fifteen minutes how long it took them to get to sleep and how long they slept. Only about one-fourth of the insomniacs came that close. Regardless of what the sleep machines said, the insomniacs had ex-perienced a much different sleep in their minds. Sleeping pills, says Roth, may not always be that effective, since they may change the sleep the body gets, the objective sleep, but not the sleep the mind remembers, the subjective part of a night's sleep.

In another test the Cincinnati group found that people were more confused about how much sleep they got after they began taking sleeping pills. This could be a dangerous effect because, if the pills not only interfere with sleep but also the way we *think* we sleep, we might end up taking a pill overdose in an attempt to correct a sleep problem that may not exist.

Not every sleep clinician you talk to is antipill. Dartmouth College psychologist and insomnia expert Dr. Peter Hauri believes the sleeping pill has some value. "You'll hear from many people that sleeping pills are just awful; they don't work," he comments. "This is because in our sleep clinics we see all the failures. We don't see the thousands of people who take the standard 50 milligrams of Dalmane, or 100 milligrams of Seconal, or whatever, are satisfied with the pills, and live to be a ripe old age. My feeling is that if a person takes one dose of something and he is satisfied, why rock the boat?" In spite of all the disagreement, it looks like if you take a single dose and take it as seldom as possible, you and your sleep should survive reasonably intact.

Maybe you've been sufficiently impressed by the story of the blackout man and by the list of things that the pills can do *to* you as well as for you. Still, you may say, "I would like to take *something* to help me sleep." What other choices do you have?

One option that may come to mind is to have a little nightcap before you turn in. The problem with getting in the habit of having little nightcaps is that before long they end up being big nightcaps and giving you big sleep problems as well. Taking alcohol as a sleep drug is essentially the same as taking barbiturates in a liquid form.

Like the barbiturates, alcohol wipes out REM sleep; it causes REM rebound; it's potentially addictive; it's especially dangerous with other sleep drugs or tranquilizers; taken long enough, it will cause insomnia and can even damage your brain's sleep mechanism; and the process of withdrawing from alcohol is exactly the same as being weaned off barbiturates.

The longer you take alcohol, the worse its rebound effect. When they are drinking, alcoholics have little or no REM sleep. Once the drinking stops, the dreams and nightmares return with a vengeance. One theory about the terrifying hallucinations of delirium tremens that some alcoholics suffer is that the hallucinations are actually waking nightmares. After years of bottling up all that REM sleep and its dreams, the brain suddenly releases them. These nightmares leak into alcoholics' days, hounding them while they're awake. Severe cases of barbiturate withdrawal have these hallucinations as well, possibly for the same reason.

As far as your body is concerned, the two drugs are identical. People who have taken a heavy dose of barbiturates literally act like drunks—staggering around, slurring their speech, showing all the exaggerated good feeling or melancholy of a person who's had one too many. According to the Consumers Union book *Licit and Illicit Drugs*, the reason for this is that alcohol and barbiturates are interchangeable in their chemical effects. Alcoholics can stop drinking completely and switch over to popping barbiturates without going through any withdrawal. Some even juggle a pill habit with a drinking habit, feeding the same addiction with two different drugs.

Basically, all you need to remember about alcohol as a sleep drug is that it will get you to sleep but it will give you an unsettled night's rest with no REM sleep, many awakenings, and erratic shifts in your sleep stages. It is identical to barbiturates in every way except one— it's a little easier to overdose with a handful of pills than with a bottle. Apart from that, having a bedtime drink is not much different than popping a sleeping pill.

As was mentioned before, some doctors avoid giving sleeping pills completely. Instead, they prescribe daytime drugs to help you at night. If it looks like your insomnia is the result of you're being too worried or anxious, your doctor may give you some tranquilizers to take during the day. Two of the most popular ones used for this purpose are Valium and Librium, members of the same drug family as the sleeping pill Dalmane. Or, if it looks like depression is at the root of your sleeplessness, you may be given an antidepressant such as Elavil, Endep, or Triavil to take before going to bed. These can work as well as, or better than, most of the sleeping pills without exposing you to the same risks because the doses are smaller.

An even safer solution is to try a little tryptophan. This is a natural protein found in a variety of foods, from peanut butter to steak. Tryptophan, or L-tryptophan as it is sometimes called, provides the raw material for a brain chemical, serotonin, which sleep researchers now know is a prime ingredient needed to switch on the sleep centers in the brain. In an average day you eat about one-half to two grams of tryptophan in your food, and you may have noticed the tryptophan effect, a drowsiness that follows a high-protein meal such as one with steak as the main course.

At Boston State Hospital, sleep researcher Dr. Ernest Hartmann found that by compacting all this tryptophan into a single, gram-sized dose—about the amount you'd get from eating a pound of steak—he could produce a mild, natural-acting sleeping pill. In a typical experiment a group of people who drank tryptophan-spiked milkshakes fell asleep twice as quickly as usual.

Encouraged by experiments like this, some sleep clinics have been using tryptophan on insomniac patients, with some good results. Montefiore Hospital sleep clinicians in New York were able to help one young stockbroker recover from a ten-month bout with insomnia and the slump in business that came with it. "It can be an impressive drug," says Montefiore's Dr. Pollok, "but it's not a drug to be used for the rest of your life. One cannot recommend it for general use, but I think it does have a certain limited place in treating insomnia."

Even here the reviews are mixed. "Frankly, I haven't had very good luck with it," another sleep clinician told me, "and I've tried it many times. Now I use it as a temporary expedient if a patient demands a pill. Sometimes I just give it to him to keep him happy until I complete my workup."

So far, the evidence is that tryptophan may work for mild cases of insomnia, but not for the serious, long-lasting type that is likely to turn up in a sleep clinic. Tryptophan also appears to be a safe drug. Doctors in Great Britain have had some success using it as a mild antidepressant and report that even in large doses it does their patients no harm.

Here in the United States tryptophan is still considered an experimental drug, but in spite of that you can buy it on the open market. You won't find it in your drug store, but in your local health food store, probably in the vitamin section. The Food and Drug Administration has classified tryptophan as a food, not a drug, since it is now available in approximately the same concentrations in tablet form that you would find in food form. You'll most likely find it labeled as L-tryptophan, and you will also find it very expensive. One check of a health food store turned up a bottle of thirty .66-gram-size mocha-colored tablets, enough for about fifteen nights, that sold for ten dollars. This is a pretty steep price to pay for a night's sleep, even when compared to prescription pills. You can get twenty-five nights' worth of chloral hydrate pills, for example, for about three dollars.

You could save yourself the money and go straight to the food source itself for your dose of tryptophan. Among the edibles that rate high in this protein are: tuna fish, liver, steak, hamburger, pork chops, chicken, turkey, peanuts, peanut butter, beans, and dairy products like cheese, cottage cheese, and that old home remedy for sleep, the glass of warm milk.

If you don't happen to be hungry, there is one other drug you could try, and it's likely that you won't even have to go out and buy it. You probably already have the drug in your medicine cabinet. "Aspirin," suggests Dr. Peter Hauri. "It works very nicely." Some insomniacs, he says, have found it helpful as a mild sleeping pill. No studies have been done on why it works, but one theory is that aspirin raises the level of the sleep chemical, serotonin, in your brain by dissolving previously indigestible tryptophan found in your bloodstream into a form the brain can use. More tryptophan rushing into the brain's sleep center eventually means more serotonin, and more serotonin means you get sleepy faster. As sleeping pills go, aspirin is hard to beat. It's cheaper than the tryptophan tablets, safer than prescription drugs, and a lot more effective than any over-the-counter drug you're likely to buy. If you want to take a pill, it's not such a bad choice.

This, then, is the lineup of drugs you have to choose from today: the useless but dangerous over-the-counter drugs; the useful but short-winded and dangerous prescription drugs; the risky nonprescription drug alcohol; the gentle but weak tryptophan; and the old stand-by, aspirin. If the drug laws change in the near future, you may also see added to the list one more drug, a drug once very popular with doctors in the last century. It is a natural substance made from plants once cultivated on special farms in the South and Midwest and was a medicine officially recognized by the U.S. government as recently as 1942. Before it was banned, it was sold as a liquid elixir in most every neighborhood drugstore and was known to be, among other things, a powerful but safe sleep-inducing drug. It is still used, unofficially and illegally, in a slightly different form as a sleep drug or tranquillizer, among other things. Its official drug listing name back in 1947 was *extractum cannabis,* and of course we know it as marijuana.

According to Dr. Sidney Cohen, an expert on the drug and professor of psychiatry at UCLA, *cannabis sativa* is regaining some of the status it lost when it became a popular street drug and is now the focus of a number of serious studies designed to explore its medical potential. Most of the attention now is on THC (for delta-9-tetrahydrocannabinol), believed to be the major active ingredient in *cannabis.* So far, indications are that it may have possible value: alleviating the nauseating side effects of cancer treatments; reducing eye pressure in glaucoma victims; giving moderate breathing relief to asthma sufferers; acting as an antibiotic, as a pain reliever, as a mild sedative, and as a sleep-inducer. Who knows, maybe ten years from now doctors will be prescribing *extractum cannabis* for insomnia in amounts that today would cost the patient a stiff fine or some time in prison. Stranger things have happened.

5.
The Cure

It was 3:00 A.M. Suzanne's eyelids had jammed themselves open and showed no inclination to shut again. The old familiar struggle with insomnia had started. She lay there, quietly at first, waiting for sleep to come back. More time passed, more shifting and flopping around in bed. "Enough is enough," she finally thought and climbed out of bed to get her sleep medicine. She headed not for her medicine cabinet, but her refrigerator. That's where she kept her guaranteed, surefire, unpatented cure for insomnia—a bowl of cherries.

She opened the door and took out six and ate them one at a time in a slow, ritualistic way, carefully chewing each and savoring its flavors and juices. As she finished one, she'd pop the pit into the wastebasket and begin eating the next cherry, repeating the same ritual. By the time the sixth pit hit the bottom of the wastebasket, she felt calmer, more relaxed. She knew she had it beaten. She clicked off the kitchen light and headed for the bedroom. Within five minutes she was sound asleep.

Practically anything can work when it comes to overcoming insomnia. Although most people don't realize it, there are many alternatives to the overkill of the sleeping pill that can work just as well and a lot more safely. If you have the right attitude, you can seduce your body and brain to sleep with nothing more lethal than a bing cherry. All it takes is finding the right trick or combination of tricks. It's not as simple as taking a few pills, but it's a lot less dangerous.

To start, your best sleep medicine is always preventive medicine. It is possible to stop much of your insomnia before it starts by the way you handle your daytime. Whether you realize it or not, your sleep problems at night start long before your head hits your pillow. Too often you get yourself moving at such high mental speeds that when the time to sleep comes, you can't slow down fast enough. As a result, you go skidding right on by sleep and crash head-on into another night of insomnia.

According to Dr. Hans Selye, the one man most responsible for modern medicine's concept of stress, a frenzied day is probably one of the most common causes of everyday insomnia. To counter sleep interference that may leak into your night, he has what he calls his basic recipe for a good night's sleep.

The first part is not to overreact to the routine stresses that are part of your daily schedule. Every stress is an action that gets an appropriate reaction. In your body, this reaction is in the form of the chemical kick of adrenalin which speeds up your system like an amphetamine. The more intensely you react, the higher the dose of this body drug. For example, if you start getting obsessed with worry when a bill arrives in the mail or your boss asks for a report to be done on 4:30 on a Friday afternoon, you could be pumping a huge dose of this natural stimulant into your body, and it might still be there at bedtime. As a result, you may want to sleep but may also find you are much too alert to rest. If you've gotten to this point, you're in rough shape. All you can do is wait for all those natural-made amphetamines to clear from your body. And that waiting means insomnia, and insomnia becomes one more stress to an overworked, and now sleep-starved body which you are going to have to force through another day of work. The next night, even more weary and overworked, you're going to be faced with the beginning of a vicious cycle if you still can't get to sleep.

Before you get to that point, or even if you're already there, you should take the time to figure out how you can pare down your daytime stress. Some of it of course is unavoidable and comes with your job and daily living; but there are ways to minimize the pressures and to get your work done and not be left with an overload of natural stimulants rushing through your system. This is where the second part of Dr. Selye's antistress recipe comes in. Don't overwork yourself into a rut, with no variety, no breaks in your routine. If you do, you may find it hard to shut your mind off when it's time to sleep, and that work which obsessed you all day is going to come back to haunt you at night.

Since much of the work rut comes from spending too much time on daily trivia, map out your daily priorities and make sure they get done first. Everything else should be made to fit around them. This gives more structure to your time and gives you more control over it as well. Set your priorities well in advance—the day before, or at least the night before. Try any system that suits you: listing them in order of importance, in priority categories (high, medium, low), whatever appeals to your sense of order.

Also schedule your work realistically. You know from past experience how much you can get done by 5:00 P.M. Build in some breathing space or some emergency time into your schedule to give you some flexibility. Don't trap yourself by planning out a work load you can't carry. If you do, you'll be digging yourself deeper into your work rut.

Your problem may not be that your schedule is too tight, but that it's too flexible. When someone makes a demand on your time, you automatically bump those priority jobs you had so carefully lined up, take on more than you can handle, and get nothing done. Being too ready to accommodate others can throw any schedule into total chaos and put you in the rut of having to play catch-up all the time. If you can, learn to negotiate for your time—it's one of the irreplaceables in your life. Try to get the other person to see your priorities. ("Of course I can pick up your coat at the cleaner's. I'll just cancel my lunch with the governor" is always surefire.)

If you end up taking on too much work, you know that you'll find yourself back on that treadmill you're trying to avoid. You'll hate yourself for being so compliant and will lie awake most of the night worrying about all the work that didn't get done that day.

Rehearse for those times when someone springs a surprise job on you. It never hurts to have a few prepared responses ready—ranging from the old favorite, "Let me check my calendar" to "Excuse me, I think I hear gunfire"—if only to give you time to evaluate the request.

Have a pattern of thinking ready for these situations to give you a few seconds of breathing room to make a decision and frame an answer you won't later regret. Basically, if you can get in the habit of letting your first thought be, "Is it important enough for me to throw off my schedule," instead of the self-destructive "How will I ever do this?" you can be better prepared for the unexpected.

Get yourself ready for some of the routine stresses of your life by rehearsing them in your mind. The army trains its crack troops this way; there's no reason why you shouldn't adopt the method. Project yourself into one of your typical crisis work situations—an impending deadline, coordinating some mammoth project, a showdown meeting with your child's teacher. Run through the scene in your mind while you are still relaxed and distant from it. Plan your actions and reactions coolly. If thinking about meeting that deadline makes your palms sweat, stop, relax a bit, and start the mental rehearsal all over. Do this enough and you will be ready to handle the actual situation much more easily and suffer less as well.

The last bit of information Dr. Selye has to offer is to build in some variety into your day to keep from getting in a work rut. A change of pace will help take some of the tension out of your day and offer a kind of safety valve for all the pressure that's been building up. Use whatever diversion suits your personality and schedule best, whether it's relaxing with your favorite soap opera in the afternoon or going out and jogging a few miles. Some "high-power" types find that taking short catnaps, for twenty minutes or less, helps. This is what got Lyndon Johnson through a grueling day's work when he was president. You should remember that while this is a good antiinsomnia precaution, it is not a good habit to keep if you already have insomnia. Napping tends to drain off some of that fatigue that may help you get back to your old sleep schedule.

If you don't have any pressure valve built into your day, install one. Start just by practicing how to slow down and take it easy. If you commute to work, give yourself an extra ten minutes in the morning so you won't be rushed to catch your bus or train. Try doing something else other than work as you commute—read a book, plan the ideal vacation, do the crossword puzzle in the paper. When you can afford it, think SLOW: decelerate your walking speed; force yourself to slow down your eating pace by using the old diet trick of setting down your fork between bites; or repeat to yourself what other people say. That will make you a better listener and a less frantic person.

You have to know when to put on the brakes, so you can slow down in time to get to sleep. If you do any work at home, one of the most common traps you can fall into is to keep at it right up until bedtime. What happens when you climb into bed is usually that your mind, fresh from working, is racing away. Under these circumstances sleep may take hours to arrive. What is an even worse habit than working before bedtime is to work *in* bed. It's an antisleep habit and runs counter to the whole purpose of the bed and the bedroom. If you do a lot of work at home, you have to give yourself a time cushion between when you work and when you sleep. I don't care how busy your day is; that cushion is there if you really want it.

The late Hubert Humphrey, for example, knew the value of this time cushion idea. Even during the most hectic days of his presidential campaigning he always insisted on having an hour to himself at the end of the day to do anything he wanted. No matter what time he finished campaigning, at day's end his work stopped and he took his hour before bedtime. This time was sacred. Except for the most extreme emergencies, no one could interrupt. He never spent it in any spectacular way—usually just watching a late-night movie, reading, or talking with his family. But the important thing was that he used the time the way he wanted, as an oasis of peace in the midst of the frenzy of campaigning.

If you're still looking for a specific daytime pressure valve, one fad that might be worth following is jogging. Not only does it offer the frequently advertised advantages of being cheap (all you really need are the shoes), easy (even for the uncoordinated), and beneficial for the heart, lungs, and body in general, but now it looks like it also offers some other special benefits that make it appealing as an anti-insomnia tactic. Research done by psychiatrists at both the University of Virginia and the University of Wisconsin found that a steady regimen of jogging relieves what is generally one of insomnia's chief symptoms, mild depression.

University of Wisconsin psychiatrist Dr. John Greist said jogging worked as well as short-term psychotherapy on the mildly depressed. Instead of talking to their therapist, Greist's depressed patients ran with him. Their only instructions were to avoid thinking of their

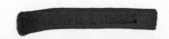

problems and instead focus on the rhythms of their breathing and their feet hitting the ground. After ten weeks of running three days a week, the patients found that most of their depression had cleared. In similar research, Dr. Robert Brown at the University of Virginia saw improvement among 800 students who regularly ran a total of three hours per week for three months.

Some possible reasons why jogging works so well, they say, is that it improves your self-image, gives you a sense of achievement, and gives you an outlet for anger and anxiety which, if turned in on yourself, can cause depression. If you plan to jog, but until now have restricted your exercise to walking from the car to the house, it might be wise to have a medical checkup and get a doctor's advice before you take the plunge, especially if you are in your mid-thirties or older. And, to minimize the shock to your body, start slowly.

If you decide to do any exercise as part of an antiinsomnia program, schedule your workout time for later in the day, not in the morning. According to Dartmouth sleep expert Dr. Peter Hauri, studies he and other experts have conducted show that any steady exercise does help you sleep if you do it late in the afternoon or early evening. Running in the morning, for example, may give you stronger legs and do wonders for your heart and lungs, but it won't help you sleep. The sleep-inducing effects have usually faded by the time you're ready for bed. Exercising very late in the evening, on the other hand, within an hour or two of bedtime, can have the opposite effect, arousing your whole system so that it becomes impossible for you to get any rest. One last exercise warning from Dr. Hauri: don't try to use exercise on a one-time basis, like a sleeping pill. It's been proven that one day of any kind of intense physical activity doesn't do anything to help your sleep at night, and it may even keep you up with all the aches and pains from overworked muscles.

As you move closer to your bedtime, you should be more conscious of what to avoid if you're having trouble sleeping or if you want to keep your nights insomnia-free. The first piece of advice all sleep experts offer is never to nap during the day, or at least not after six in the evening. Napping too late in the day diminishes your sleep appetite and will delay your bedtime.

Also watch your caffeine intake. As a general rule, have your last cup of coffee, tea, hot cocoa, or cola drink at least two hours before

bedtime or, if you want to be safe, four hours. Your body starts feeling the stimulating effect of the caffeine between thirty minutes to an hour after you drink it. The peak of stimulation comes two to four hours after you take it, but the wide-awake effects can linger for several hours afterward.

Caffeine is probably one of the most forgotten causes of insomnia. If you took the time to keep a detailed sleep log, you may have been surprised to find out how much caffeine you drink in a typical day. One of the problems with coffee is that people think of it as a social drink, never as a drug; but, according to a study done by doctors at Stanford University's Medical School, a daily habit of five cups or more can bring with it a genuine dependence on caffeine. A daily habit of seven to ten cups is almost a guarantee of sleep problems. (Caffeine, however, is not a tremendously dangerous drug. By one estimate, a lethal dose is one gram, about the amount of caffeine in seventy to a hundred cups of coffee.)

To get an idea of what your caffeine intake is, you could compare it to something a little easier to visualize, such as the caffeine pills you can buy in the drugstore under the brand name of NoDoz. Each tablet is 100 milligrams of caffeine, roughly equivalent to the average dose in one five-ounce cup of brewed coffee. (One cup contains anywhere from 80 to 120 milligrams of the drug.) That same cup filled with instant coffee has about three-quarters as much caffeine, while a cup of tea or cocoa will give you half as much. And if you drink a twelve-ounce can of cola drink, you're also imbibing the ice-cold liquid equivalent of one caffeine tablet. Don't forget, coffee may not be your only caffeine source.

It's conceivable that you're one of those rare people who sleeps better after a cup of coffee. Medical studies done in Canada and West Germany found that a cup of coffee or strong cup of tea taken at bedtime actually helps some of the elderly sleep more soundly. You can risk part of a night's sleep if you want to see if you fit into that rare category, but the odds are you don't.

Caffeine isn't the only drug that can give you insomnia. If you are now taking any kind of prescription drug and have trouble sleeping, you might ask your doctor if it's possible the drug is keeping you awake. Some diet pills and antidepressant drugs are stimulants as well, so it's conceivable that while you're losing weight you may be losing sleep as well. Decongestants used in nonprescription cold medicines also have stimulating side effects and can keep you up at night. Read the package warnings when you buy them.

Each of these drugs by itself can make a real dent in a normal night's sleep, but in combination with each other they may be devastating. Take Andy for example. He went to his doctor complaining about insomnia and wanted a pill to make it go away. Instead of reaching for his prescription pad, the physician started asking Andy a few questions about his daily habits. He found out that Andy worked as a cashier in an Italian restaurant, a job he liked because his meals were free. Unfortunately for his waistline, he loved Italian food. Between eating his way through the restaurant's menu and pushing the buttons on the cash register as his sole exercise, he was zooming up toward the 300-pound mark.

His weight problem had gotten so bad he turned to diet pills to help him lose pounds. He also mentioned in the interview that he drank six cups of coffee each day. It turned out it wasn't exactly coffee he was drinking, but espresso. And not in those little thimble-sized demitasse cups, but in regular-sized coffee cups. So, between the heavy doses of espresso and the diet pills, he had enough stimulants moving in him to keep three people awake. The doctor's prescription was simply to cut way back on his espresso habit, drink none after six o'clock at night, and to go on a pill-free diet. Within a week Andy's sleep had returned to normal.

Another habit that can effect your sleep involves *when* you eat. In general, allow about three hours between your last big meal of the day and bedtime. That will give your digestive system plenty of time to absorb all the food and relax. To operate at peak efficiency, your stomach has to be "awake," otherwise you might be unpleasantly awakened in the middle of the night by a bad spell of heartburn, as a sleepy, sluggish digestive tract tries to handle that nine o'clock meal or pepperoni pizza snack.

Like many rules, this one has an exception. Sleep experts have found that people sleep less well and are more prone to insomnia when dieting. Tests with animals showed that the less they ate, the less they slept. Doctors have also noticed that hospital patients who have lost weight often complain of waking up many times during the night and in general sleeping poorly. This has been especially marked among those suffering from anorexia nervosa, in which patients, usually women, almost starve themselves to death in their obsession over losing weight.

The reason for this diet-insomnia connection isn't clear, but one plausible theory is that it's a built-in survival mechanism. A hungry human or animal has to be awake to find food. Insomnia in this case is the body's way of making us stay up until we get our three square meals.

If you think your diet may be losing you sleep as well as pounds, or even if you're not on a diet but are plagued by early-morning awakenings, you might want to try a *light* prebedtime snack or beverage that will keep your stomach from stirring you in the middle of the night. A warm glass of milk (make it skim) is a good choice for a number of reasons. It is loaded with the natural sleep-inducing chemical tryptophan. Its warmth should help to soothe and relax you, and the process of digesting it will draw some blood away from an alert brain, helping you unwind a little. For variety's sake you might try flavoring it with Ovaltine (not cocoa—that contains caffeine).

You might try other warm liquids if you're not a warm milk person. Herb teas can be pleasant bedtime drinks and nonthreatening ones as well, since they have no caffeine. Some people find a peppermint or a camomile tea particularly soothing. And if you'd like something a bit more substantial but nonfattening, you might try some cottage cheese or some tuna fish before bed. Both are low in calories and high in tryptophan.

Instead of drinking a warm liquid, try surrounding yourself with it instead. Take a hot bath about a half-hour before bedtime. Make a small production of it. Bring a book in with you. Let the heat of the water soak into your body, soothing the tension and aches. The warm water will not only relax your muscles, it should relax your mind by drawing blood to the outside of your body and away from your brain.

But all those daily precautions—those miles you jogged, the warm milk, and the warm baths—won't do a thing for you if you don't observe the most basic of antiinsomnia rules: *have a set bedtime ritual.* At the very least it should include:

- A regular bedtime
- A regular wakeup time

- A bedroom that's been "prepared" for sleep
- A presleep routine that helps you gradually break your ties with the day

Sleep is a regular, timed part of your body's twenty-four-hour cycle. If you're going to enjoy its benefits, you have to respect the rhythmic part of its nature. You can follow a reasonably regular bedtime without being rigid. Try not to vary when you go to bed by more than a half-hour at night. Your sleep clock needs that reassurance.

What also helps keep that sleep time regular is having a set wakeup time at the other end of the night. For most people, that isn't a problem, since they have a job or school or some pressing obligation to get them out of bed; but people who are retired, or are not working for one reason or another sometimes fall into the trap of not following a steady morning routine. They may stay in bed later on some days than others, continually varying their rising time. The result is, at the end of the day they're not sleepy when they go to bed at their usual time. And they may lie in bed in misery, never making the connection between their insomnia and their careless morning habits. If you're guilty of this, create a morning ritual that will help get you going. It could be as mundane as starting your morning coffee or going out after the paper to taking an early-morning walk or jog, if you are so inclined. But you have to have some kind of a routine.

If you have an apple, a plane ticket to Paris, and know how to find the Arc de Triomphe, you can also try the solution prescribed for Alexandre Dumas (Père). To get him to follow regular sleep hours, Dumas's doctor ordered him out of bed early enough to make it to the base of the Arc de Triomphe by 7 A.M., where the famous writer was to stand and eat an apple. (Although it probably made the Parisian fruit vendors happy, there's no record of how well it worked.) The point is, your body needs the reassurance that comes with a set, predictable schedule in order for your sleep clock to work smoothly.

Is your bedroom prepared for sleep? University of Iowa psychologist Dr. Thomas Borkovec found that one thing all good sleepers have in common is that their bedrooms are efficiently organized clusters of sleep cues. They're set up to be as sleep-inducing as possible. They have certain noise and light levels, and certain room temperatures. Good sleepers also have certain people with whom they sleep. When these cues are disrupted—for example, when you are in a strange bed-room, or if your bedmate is absent—sleep problems often come.

If you take the time to look around, you can probably single out the important sleep cues in your bedroom. You no doubt have a favorite pillow or pillows, a favorite side of the bed, even a favorite kind of mattress. Maybe you also like to sleep with the window open, letting lots of cold air and noise fill the room. Or you might prefer a warm, snug room with the windows sealed shut and the shades drawn. You might even have emergency back-up cues for those nights when sleep doesn't come as smoothly as you'd like it to. Comedian George Burns told one reporter that on the nights when he couldn't sleep, he climbed into the bed his late wife Gracie used once she developed a heart condition. When he did this, he found he slept like a baby.

For years sleep researchers have been trying to figure out which bedroom conditions work for purely psychological reasons—your teddy bear, for example, is not going to help anyone else—and which have some truly objective sleep value for everyone.

They've discovered, for example, that you don't even need the bed unless you have some specific medical problem, such as a bad back. In theory at least, you should be able to sleep on almost anything. Some South American Indians sleep dangling in hammocks; some Japanese get their rest lying on the floor. In Europe, many people sleep with the head slightly elevated, reminiscent of the days when it was thought that the only healthy way to sleep was sitting up. In space, astronauts slept quite well while floating in zero gravity. Here in the United States, people sleep on lumpy, sagging mattresses, on brick-hard mattresses, on sloshing water beds, and on inflatable beds. Pillows are variously hard, soft, thin or thick, stuffed with feathers or synthetic materials (such as Dacron fibers), or foam for those with allergies. With the exception of a very hard surface, such as the floor, which, not surprisingly, sleep researchers found causes a restless night's sleep, all the bedding equipment available seems to work equally well. Mostly it comes down to how much you really believe in that bed, mattress, or pillow.

There are some changes you might make if you are concerned about making the bed a better playground. Sex expert Dr. Alex Comfort suggests buying a hard mattress—hard as you can stand without inter-fering with sleep—and also four pillows, two soft ones for sleeping, and two firm ones for lovemaking. Any other bedside equipment you wish to add to improve the atmosphere or your performance is up to you.

So far, only two parts of your bedroom environment seem to make any measurable difference in how well you might sleep. They are: temperature and noise. Various experiments have shown that certain animals have their own ideal sleep temperatures. The rat gets its best rest at around 90 degrees Fahrenheit, while the cat seems to prefer a slightly cooler temperature of 72 degrees. Although no one has yet figured out what the ideal temperature is for humans, sleep researchers do know that the warmer the bedroom temperature, the more nightmares and unpleasant dreams you are likely to have. The higher the temperature climbs above 75 degrees Fahrenheit (24 Celsius), the more restless and shallow sleep becomes. Probably because individual body thermostats and sensitivity to cold vary, there is no ideal temperature for everyone. How you sleep in a certain temperature can be as much a matter of your attitude as where the mercury sits. "The person who throws open the bedroom window during 50-degree spring nights and sleeps like a baby," says one sleep expert, "may wake and turn up the dial on his electric blanket if the room gets that cold in the winter."

The other big environmental enemy of sleep is noise. Again, absolutes are difficult to find, because people's sensitivity to sound varies. Sound sensitivity also varies according to the stage of sleep you are in, your sex, and your age, as well, of course, as where you live. The same sound that wakes you in the early part of the night when you are still in shallow sleep may go completely unnoticed later on when you are at deep sleep levels. Sound tests have also shown that women will awaken more quickly than men to the same aircraft noise, while the elderly, especially those seventy and over, are all more noise sensitive, probably because their sleep is shallow for most of the night.

As you probably already know, you can train yourself to awaken to certain sounds. One friend of mine described how, when he was stationed in Vietnam, he could routinely sleep through the usual nightly racket of friendly fire around his base camp: machine-gun fire, the night-long thumping sound of mortars, and the big guns of heavy artillery nearby. He was also able to awaken at the first, faint sound of enemy mortar fire. Mortar attacks were a weekly event, so he learned to sharpen his ear quickly. Even though the mortar sound was actually fainter than the sounds immediately around him, his "radar," as he called it, always picked it out and woke him before the first shells hit the camp. He never explained how he was able to do this. "My only guess," he says, "is that I was highly motivated not to get blown up."

Being familiar with a noise will not always make you immune to its sleep-robbing effects. Noise-sleep studies have found that once a sound passes above the 60-decibel level—about equal to the noise generated by a trailer truck rumbling down your street—most people will wake up or at least be disturbed in their sleep. Night noises can come from anywhere, but one very common source could be your garbage cans— not because of the raccoon or neighborhood dog that occasionally knocks them over, but because of the people who make those regular early morning pickups.

According to the Environmental Protection Agency's Office of Noise Abatement and Control, on a typical night in the United States garbage trucks all over the country are responsible for 34 million "sleep disturbances," to use the agency's terms. In hearings on the topic, the agency heard stories like the one told by a local Chicago politician. His constituents would call him early in the morning and then stick their phones out the window so he could hear the racket the trucks were making. The EPA is now trying to make it law that no whining, humming, "truck-mounted-solid-waste-compactor" makes more than 75 decibels of noise.

Airports also cause their share of sleep problems, largely because of the 120-decibel-level sonic booms and generally high noise level created by jet aircraft. One survey of people who had lived near Los Angeles International Airport for at least six years found that, while the people claimed they were used to the nightly air traffic noise, sleep monitoring tests done in their own homes showed that they had less deep sleep, more shallow sleep, and more brief awakenings at night than people who lived in a quieter part of the city.

In general, it looks like you can adapt your sleep to most noises if they are part of the background of a typical night's sleep; but this adaptive ability will only carry you so far if the noise is loud enough. Your sleep can suffer in subtle ways you may not even be aware of. For that reason, you should take special care to provide some kind of sound insulation in your bedroom (you will find some specific suggestions later in this chapter). Don't underestimate the power of noise to ruin sleep, even when you're "used to it."

Your bedroom may be ready for sleep, but are you? Do you have a sleep ritual or is it an insomnia ritual? Loosely speaking, a sleep ritual is any habit or series of habits that gradually leads you away from the frenzy of the day to the quiet and rest of sleep. As part of the ritual, stress expert Hans Selye recommends any sort of task that ends in a successful resolution. (He himself swims and exercises for a half-hour before bedtime.) For some people this may involve laying out the clothes they plan to wear the next day. For others, like newscaster Barbara Walters, it consists of making a list of priority things to do the next day.

For still others the ritual can be much more elaborate. Actress Gloria Swanson gets ready for bed by stretching out on the floor with a thick Japanese quilt, taking great care to align her body on a magnetic north–south axis (her head toward the north, her feet toward the south) to be in harmony with the earth's magnetic field. The belief that aligning your body according to the earth's magnetic poles helps bring sleep dates back at least to the nineteenth century, when one of its most avid believers was the author Charles Dickens. Dickens always carried a compass with him, and whenever he came to a new hotel room one of the first things he would do would be to shift the bed around until it was pointing north and south. He was especially meticulous about how he lay in the bed. He had to be dead center in it, his body equidistant from the top, bottom, and sides.

So far, there is no firm scientific justification for this magnetic-wave theory of sleep, although it is conceivable that we have some sensitivity to magnetic field shifts. We already know that lower animals do. Worms and some mollusks are sensitive to it, and so are homing pigeons, who find their way back to the roost by magnetic waves. And, according to body rhythm expert Gay Gaer Luce, people have had some unusual experiences involving the earth's magnetic poles. Men who have spent time at the South Pole have been known to lose their deepest stage of sleep, stage 4, while there. In one case the person's stage-4 sleep didn't return until a year after he had left the pole. But so far no one has managed to make a direct connection between the

north-south magnetic theory and getting to sleep. Until they do, you
may as well save your compass for your camping trips.

Probably the most popular of presleep rituals, next to watching
Johnny Carson's monologue, is reading. I have one friend, for example, who flexes his college French by reading mysteries by the
master of the form, Georges Simenon. You might also use the time
to nibble away at the 800-page best-seller you bought but never got a
chance to read, or, if you'd like to kill two birds with one stone by
getting some culture as well as a little sleep, try one of the fifteen
most boring classics, compiled in the *Book of Lists* from a Columbia
University Press survey. They are, in order of ennui:

1. *Pilgrim's Progress*, by John Bunyan
2. *Moby Dick*, by Herman Melville
3. *Paradise Lost*, by John Milton
4. *Faerie Queene*, by Edmund Spenser
5. *Life of Samuel Johnson*, by James Boswell
6. *Pamela*, by Samuel Richardson
7. *Silas Marner*, by George Eliot
8. *Ivanhoe*, by Sir Walter Scott
9. *Don Quixote*, by Miguel de Cervantes
10. *Faust*, by Johann Wolfgang von Goethe
11. *War and Peace*, by Leo Tolstoy
12. *Remembrance of Things Past*, by Marcel Proust
13. *Das Kapital*, by Karl Marx
14. *Vanity Fair*, by William Makepeace Thackeray
15. *The Mill on the Floss*, by George Eliot

The big advantage of having any kind of bedtime reading, dull or
otherwise, is that it makes a big part of your sleep ritual portable, so
you can find it easier to rest no matter where you are.

"But I don't have *any* sleep ritual!" you may say. If you usually get
to sleep at night, you probably do. The next time you are getting ready
for bed, slow down a little and watch yourself. You'll find you are
doing certain things in a specific order. You'll probably find for example that you may only brush your teeth after you've dressed, or
undressed, for bed. You may turn out certain lights, check the doors

and windows in your home, let the cat in (or out), or, if you are a religious person, you may say some prayers—all in a certain predictable, set order before you go to sleep. It's a ceremony you may not notice, but, if you have any doubt it exists, just ask your spouse, lover, or roommate. He or she can probably give a detailed account of exactly how you spend your last few minutes of wakefulness every night.

As one last part of the sleep ritual, you probably also have a favorite bed position. According to psychiatrist Dr. Samuel Dunkell, who covers the body language of sleepers in his book *Sleep Positions*, there is a certain choreography to the way we lie in the bed during a night's sleep. Generally, says Dunkell, everyone has two bed postures: the Alpha position, and the Omega position. The Alpha position is the one you assume as you lie there awake but relaxed, ready to settle into the first stages of sleep. As you sense sleep coming on, you shift into your Omega position, the one you'll keep for most of your serious sleeping.

If you don't have a sleep position, Dr. Robert Van de Castle of the University of Virginia sleep lab suggests that you cultivate one. Just let your body settle into whatever feels naturally comfortable. You may have to experiment a little, lying on your back, sides, and stomach before you find what you like, but eventually you'll find it. According to Dr. Dunkell, one of the most comfortable positions is the *swastika*, so-called because the body adopts a kind of crude imitation of the infamous broken-cross design. In this position the sleeper lies on his stomach, one arm extended above his head and the other bent and extended below the shoulder. The legs are bent as though the sleeper is running.

What if, in spite of all your precautions, you start getting that creeping feeling that there's a struggle going on inside you between sleep and waking, and sleep is losing?

The first thing to do is try not to panic, or at least try not to panic too badly. If you're prepared to lie there with that "Oh well, here goes another night's sleep down the tubes" attitude, that's exactly what is likely to happen. What you have to do is go on the attack and try to force insomnia out of your mind.

This is not the same thing as forcing yourself to sleep. Unless you have a yogi's powers of self-control, there is no way you can induce sleep the way you can induce wakefulness. What will usually happen when you try that is you will get the opposite effect. Concentrating on sleep draws you into a vicious cycle of worrying about insomnia and generating insomnia because of the worrying. If you're having trouble getting to sleep, the trick is to concentrate on something else to beat it.

Try everyone's favorite bedroom distraction, sex. There is a lot to recommend it. It's healthy exercise (burns up about 150 calories). It's a good way to reaffirm your relationship. It's fun. And it's one of the best sleep medicines around. Catherine the Great of Russia, one of history's famous insomniacs, recommended having sex at least six times a day. Studies of sex as a sleep inducer have shown that it works well for both men and women, although men seem to benefit a little more from it. They seem to get more deep sleep after a session of love-making. If your bed partner is awake and willing, sex is always worth a try. Even if you don't get to sleep, it beats staring at the ceiling.

If that doesn't work, try it again. Then try some mind games. Two Harvard psychologists, Richard Davidson and Gary Schwartz, studied one traditional sleep-inducing method, counting sheep, and found that it actually works. It blocks out troublesome brain interference the way military electronics equipment can jam radio broadcasts. Their explanation is based on something called split-brain theory. It is generally believed that our brain is divided into two halves, each of which handles a special kind of mental work. The right side takes care of most of our more artistic functions, since it handles the way we process such things as images (paintings) and sounds (music). The left side is more practical. It is in charge of rational work, such as logic and math. Sheep counting blocks both these brain hemispheres by providing distracting images (the jumping sheep) and a rational distraction (in the form of the sheep counting).

You can count sheep if you wish, and you may bore yourself to sleep. I always have trouble with the sheep method because I can never remember what they look like. (Do they have horns or don't they? Are they white, gray? Is their wool curly, or long and shaggy?) What keeps coming to mind is not a neat picture of sheep hopping a fence one by one, but herds of sheep stupidly wandering around, colliding with each other, bleating, and staring at me with blank, dumb eyes. If the sheep trick doesn't work either, there are others.

Think of a brand new blackboard, completely clean. A deep, dark, velvety black. Pick up a piece of chalk and, as slowly as possible, draw a big white "3" on it in sweeping, lazy curves, studying the lines as you make them. When that 3 is done, write another one next to it, in the same slow way. Continue doing this the length of the blackboard until you get to sleep. A variation on this is to count backward slowly, starting from 100. Write 100 on your blackboard. Erase it and write 99. Erase it and write 98, and so on. Keep on going down until you can't go any farther.

Fantasies can also give you the same effect, especially if they are exclusively bedtime fantasies and part of your presleep night. One you might try is to think about everything you've always wanted to buy. Give yourself one million dollars, or five million, or ten million—whatever you think will pay the bill. Now start running down the list of what you would get with it—the cars, houses, clothes, jewels, or other playthings you would get; the people you'd give the money to (or buy out); the places you would visit; the parties you'd throw. It's your money; spend it any way you want. Or you might have a dream house in mind. Map out your floor plan and pick out your architectural design. Start building it, very slowly. If you get done, furnish the rooms, carefully, lovingly, one at a time. When your dream house gets built, take off on your ideal around-the-world trip. Whatever you think may work, try it.

If you're a word freak, mind games may help. Some find that composing palindromes (such as "Madam, I'm Adam," "A man, a plan, a canal—Panama," or Napoleon's palindrome, "Able was I 'ere I saw Elba") is a handy distraction. Others work their way through the alphabet, rhyming word pairs: anchor-banker, able-cable, abortion-distortion, academy-epitome . . . you get the idea. Slightly more challenging is a variation of this, rhyming titles. For example, kindergarten becomes a lilliputian institution; the leader of a team of insects is a roach coach; a coffee-maker is a caffeine machine. Try not to get too carried away so you won't end up waking your bedmate for suggestions.

If mind games aren't your forte, you might try sound to help distract you from worrying about sleep. Dr. Van de Castle of the University of Virginia recommends listening to a relaxing record to help you sleep. You might be able to find a few in your record collection, or you might try some "environment" records produced for this purpose. Some recording companies have come out with a whole line of realistic recordings of soothing natural sounds, such as waves breaking on the shore, the rustling of trees, and the woodsy cricket and cicada sounds that come at dusk. If you can't find anything like this in your record shop, try the mail-order scientific equipment company Edmund Scientific Company (Dept. AD01, Edscorp Building, Barrington, NJ 08007). Their catalogue is free for the asking.

There are "white noise" machines available that are supposed to have the same effect as environment records, creating a soothing background of noise to help you sleep. They're often recommended as sleep aids not only for their monotonous hypnotic effect, but for their noise-blocking powers as well. The only problems with these machines is that for the amount of use you will get out of them they are overpriced (some cost well over $100) and they don't always seem to work that well. One sleep study with a white noise machine found that it even disrupted sleep slightly while it was in use. The advantage records have over white noise machines is that they last only a short while. If you have an automatic turntable, records will shut themselves off, leaving you and your sleep alone. Records are also a lot cheaper.

If you're not familiar with "white noise," the simplest way to find out what it sounds like is to turn on your television set and flip the selector to a blank channel (in most areas this is channel 12). Now turn up the volume. You'll hear a kind of fuzzy, hissing sound. That's it. A few years ago one newspaper recommended using a TV set as a white noise machine, by doing just this—tuning to a blank channel and turning up the volume. It also suggested covering the set with a blanket so the light wouldn't keep you awake. Some readers who followed this advice woke in the middle of the night to find their television set in flames. And one woman found that the blanket draped over the television set had trapped all the TV heat; the result was that the plastic chassis of her portable set melted like a caramel left out in the sun.

Other sounds besides music and hissing can relax you. One technique that has been tried with some success in sleep clinics uses nothing more complicated than one of those wind-up metronomes, the kind you may have once used to pace your piano scales. If you own one, set it for sixty beats per minute and place it within earshot.

Listen to it as you lie in bed, pacing your breathing (closed mouth) rhythm to its beats. You can experiment to find the system that's the most relaxing, but in the beginning you can try timing your breaths so that it takes you eight metronome beats to exhale very slowly, pause on the ninth beat, and then take eight more beats to inhale equally slowly. It would work this way. EX(two-three-four-five-six-seven)HALE. (PAUSE.) IN(two-three-four-five-six-seven)HALE. As you let your breathing settle into this rhythm, you should find yourself becoming a little more relaxed and, eventually, drowsy.

For a particularly stubborn insomnia, you might try a system devised by Northwestern University psychologist Richard R. Bootzin. It's a six-part strategy he calls "Stimulus Control Behavior Therapy," which is nothing more than a way to counter the bad habit of self-inflicted insomnia.

His six rules are as follows:

1. You can lie in the bed only if you feel sleepy.
2. Use the bed only for sleep and sex. You are not allowed to work, eat, read, or even watch television while in bed. These must all be done in some other room.
3. If you don't fall asleep within thirty minutes at the beginning of the night, get up and leave the room. Return to bed only when you feel sleepy. If sleep does not come within ten minutes of your return, get up again and leave the room.
4. Repeat step 3 as long as necessary, until sleep comes.
5. Regardless of how little you may have slept during the night, you have to get up at the same time every morning. This is to help force your sleep cycle into shape.
6. No matter how tired you feel the next day, you are not allowed to nap.

Dr. Bootzin says he has managed to cure close to two-thirds of the insomniacs he sees with this system. If you're thinking of trying it out, you should know that it can be a tough regimen to follow. Often you may get little or no sleep the first few nights and you may find it hard forcing yourself out of a warm comfortable bed into a chilly room. It does take a lot of will power, but if you want to sleep badly enough you can make it work. The principle behind it, of course, is to retrain your attitudes so that you associate the bedroom only with sleep and sex, not worries about insomnia or about work.

Those are some techniques you can try when the insomnia rises up from inside you. But what about specific problems out of your control, such as jet lag? With no preparation, it can take days for you to adjust to a new time zone, depending on how drastic the time shift was, how stubborn your body clock is, and even whether you were flying east or west. What makes the big difference in jet lag is time-zone crossing, not travel time. You could fly from the North Pole to the South Pole in a single day and, as long as you stay in the alley of the same time zone, you might feel tired from the long flight, but you would never go through the total body upset that comes with jet lag.

As travel has speeded up, so have the cruel effects of the lag: insomnia, indigestion, fuzzy thinking, and a general feeling of sluggishness. There is no way at present to avoid it completely, although for the future some drug companies are experimenting with special travelers' pills that will help reset the body clock with hormones. Until such pills appear, there are a few steps you can take to minimize your body shock.

You should know that, first of all, some body rhythms take longer than others to get into step with a new local time. For example, it can take as long as a week for the rhythm of your hormone secretions to adjust to the new schedule. It may take even two weeks for your rhythm of temperature highs (which are supposed to fall during the day) and lows (which usually come at night) to adjust. Usually, though, you'll find that your basic rhythms of sleep and your appetite will get in tune in two or three days.

There is also a slight difference in the time adjustment you go through that varies with the direction of your flight. For some reason, most travelers find it easier to get used to time change when flying west than flying east. That means that if you flew from New York to Honolulu, you would snap out of your jet lag more quickly than if you flew the same time zone distance (six hours) east to London, for example. One other variable that will affect your lag time is age. Young bodies adjust more easily. One study of Air France pilots flying the Paris-New York run found that the younger pilots showed much less time-lag fatigue than the older ones.

Whatever your age or the direction of your flight, you can anticipate some of the time changes before you leave by doing a little tinkering with your body clock. If you're flying east, say New York to London, you'll want to set your body clock ahead, because London time is six hours ahead of New York time. Three nights before takeoff, go to bed an hour later than usual. On the second night before your flight, make it two hours later, and on the night before, three hours. For flying west, turn your clock back by progressively going to bed one hour earlier on each of the three nights before flight time.

Be kind to your body while you're on the plane and during your first few days on the ground. Go easy on big meals and alcoholic drinks. They tend to put more strain on an already confused digestive system. For comfort's sake, wear loose clothes on the flight and try to get up and walk around a little to keep your circulation and muscles in tone. After you have landed, make your first day in the new time zone a slow-paced one, but also make a real effort to get in tune with local time as quickly as possible. When you've settled in your hotel, for example, get out and take a stroll. This flexes your leg muscles, which have been cramped in an airplane seat for hours, and it gets you into the local tempo. Lastly, if you have trouble sleeping that first night, don't worry. Try some of the sleep-inducing tactics mentioned in this chapter, but don't turn to sleeping pills or alcohol. Your sleep clock will come around in a day or two without artificial help.

When you can manage it, try to catch a flight that will land you at your destination around bedtime. Do your heavy long-distance traveling in the day rather than at night. Overnight flights going east, for example, usually mean a sleepless night on the airplane and landing at your destination in the morning, when everyone is alert and awake but you.

You don't have to fly to Europe to experience another maddening cause of insomnia, plain old noise. As was mentioned before, everything from garbage trucks to 747s seems bent on attacking our sleep, making our few hours of peace and quiet anything but that.

If your noise problem is only going to be temporary—a noisy hotel room or a brief spell of emergency repair work down the street—you can probably get by with earplugs. Most drugstores carry a selection of them. If you can't find any, write to Flents Products Company (Box 2109, Belden Station, Norwalk, CT 06852). This company specializes in items to cover your eyes and plug your ears: sleep masks, eye patches, and about five different kinds of earplugs. They have a small brochure that is free for the asking. Based on sound-deadening studies, probably your best choice of their stock is a disposable earplug that looks like a large clump of cotton. You simply tear off small tufts of this wad of synthetic fiber and put them in your ear. You can expect to block about 20 decibels more noise with these.

You may not realize it, but you may already have some good antinoise weapons at your disposal in the form of storm windows in the winter and your bedroom air conditioner or window fan in the summer. The storm windows set up a solid barrier to racket, while the white noise created by the fan or air conditioner blurs the racket away.

To improve on this sound protection and, incidentally, to conserve heat as well, take the time to seal the cracks around your bedroom window casements. Where air can get in, so can sound waves. They are extremely wily and will sneak into your bedroom wherever you let them. By closing up all the cracks and air leaks with caulking material, you can reduce the noise level in a room by as much as 10 decibels.

Curtains or drapes, the thicker the better, also make good noise sponges because they are porous, and therefore sound-absorbent. If you have a real problem window, you can increase the sound insulation by putting a second layer of curtains or drapes over it. The curtain material should not be solid, such as plastic or vinyl. Velvet or woven fiberglass drapes are your best choice for promoting quiet.

For defense against loud next-door neighbors whose idea of an open marriage is a screaming match at three in the morning, or the person who likes to play his entire collection of bagpipe records at sunrise, you can get some sound insulation by using a modification of the curtain approach. Wall hangings, decorative rugs, or even quilts—if you are a collector or quiltmaker—hung on the noisy wall should cut down some of the incoming racket. And if you like the bulletin-board look, you can do what Marcel Proust did to sound-proof his bedroom —put up corkboard. It should be at least an inch thick to be sound effective. Experts claim that corkboard absorbs from one-half to well over three-fourths of the sound that may come seeping through the walls.

If the upstairs neighbors are a real problem, you can always move, ask them to move, lie there and suffer, or, if you plan to stay where you are, put in a drop ceiling with acoustical tiles. Do not get the kinds of tiles that can be stapled, glued, or nailed directly to the ceiling, because they won't keep the room as quiet as the kind that are suspended. That cushion of air between the acoustical ceiling and the real ceiling helps the tiles deaden outside sounds even more.

By now you've probably guessed that curing your insomnia is not easy; it may in fact get very complicated, even frustrating. Where the cause is obvious—loud neighbors, heavy traffic noise, or a body clock temporarily askew from jet lag—the cure is usually simple and straight-forward. But when you "just can't sleep," then it becomes a trial-and-error process. As complicated as insomnia can sometimes get, you will be slightly ahead of the problem if you are guided by the following hints:

INSOMNIAC'S FIRST AID KIT

1. Pace your day with your night in mind, especially if a decent night's sleep has been eluding you.

2. Develop an exercise regimen late in the afternoon or in the early evening.

3. Leave yourself a time buffer of a half-hour or more to help you ease from your day to a night's sleep.

4. Follow a presleep ritual, or develop one if you don't have one. Be especially faithful to keeping the same bedtime and wakeup time.

5. Avoid naps during the day, and caffeine and heavy meals within two hours or less of bedtime.

6. Prepare your bedroom as a pleasant place to sleep, making sure it is dark, cool, quiet, and free of distractions.

7. Don't read, eat, or work in bed. Use your bed only for sex and sleep.

8. Avoid using sleeping pills and alcohol.

9. Don't try to force sleep. Let it happen. Try mind-game distractions to help it along.

10. If you still can't sleep, get up and do your suffering in another room, and follow the Bootzin stimulus control technique.

Or, you can buy a bowl of cherries.

6.
Unwinding

Knots. You can feel them being tied inside of you on your worst days. You get stuck in rush-hour traffic (a little overhand knot), someone sideswipes your new car (big square knot), your infant son refuses to eat and redecorates the kitchen with his food (medium-size knot), or a work project you've been sweating over for six months crumbles into dust in front of your eyes (a great big knot). By the end of the day you're one big Gordian knot that is not about to unravel by bedtime. Anger, stress, tension have all tied you up, have gotten you aroused and kept you aroused way past midnight.

Some people are lucky and manage to defuse this anger and tension before bedtime. For example, there's Janis, an ordinarily calm, easygoing housewife left with the burden of raising a family of six by herself while her husband pays the bills by working on remote oil field construction sites. What does she do on her bad days when it all gets too much? "I destroy things. I don't dare hit the kids. I'd probably kill them," she says, half-jokingly. "To date I've totalled three kitchen chairs, one set of china—settings for eight—and last week I kicked out the bottom half of our storm door."

"Why do I do it? Because I feel so good after its over. So calm."

Or there is the writer who has put more than one typewriter in its grave by beating it with his fists and feet when caught between the paralysis of writer's block and the pressure of a deadline. "It helps calm me down and break my writer's block," he says, "unfortunately it sometimes breaks the typewriter as well."

There is a therapeutic moral here. If you can figure out the way to break the hold of that tension, of all that compressed anger, your transition into sleep will be that much smoother. The problem is finding the way. Often you'll find that intense pressure or tension is strong enough to overpower many of the precautions and cures mentioned in Chapter 5. You'll have to find something a little more potent to help you relax and help you sleep. Fortunately, there are ways that get your body to work with you instead of against you, and that are as effective as tension releasers as kicking in a storm door or beating a typewriter to death—and they are much quieter and less expensive.

Probably the most commonly used method favored by sleep clinicians and other experts is Progressive Relaxation, sometimes also called the Jacobsonian Technique, after the man who devised it, physiologist Dr. Edmund Jacobson. Very simply, it is a system of methodically going through your body and, in an indirect way, squeezing tension from it by flexing and relaxing muscles in a special order. Jacobson developed the method as a way of tricking the body into unwinding. His technique uses the fact that most people naturally seem to prefer a more active state of the mind and body, and that it takes them a while to relax at the best of times. When you're tense, you may be tired, but you may also be so worked up and aroused inside that it's almost impossible for you to calm down, to start untying those knots.

What Jacobson has devised is a method that let's you satisfy your body's appetite for activity by doing something physical but which at the same time helps you uncoil. To do the exercises all you need are two things: time, about twenty to thirty minutes; and a comfortable place where you can sit or lie down.

For best results, plan your practice time a half-hour or so before you go to bed. You will follow a set format of tensing and relaxing muscles in your body, starting with your arms, and then moving on to your head and face, your neck and shoulders, your stomach, and then your buttocks, legs, and feet. To get the most out of these exercises, don't cheat; do your whole body. As you're performing the exercises, focus all your attention on the sensations of tension, and of relaxation. The point is to make you aware of your body, the tension it contains, and how soothing relaxation really feels.

The first step is to go to your relaxing place and lie down or stretch out, your arms lying loosely at your sides, palms facing down. Make sure there are no distractions in the room. Turn off any radio, television, or stereo and turn off the lights. Now close your eyes.

Take a deep breath, hold it for about five seconds. Exhale. Do this five more times. You should feel a little looser, a little more relaxed. As you're lying there peacefully, lift up your hands, slightly bending them at the wrists so the fingers are pointing at the ceiling. Concentrate on the tension in the lower arm. Notice the pull and tug of the muscles, the strain around your wrist. Hold your hands like this for about five seconds, then drop them suddenly. Notice the feeling of release, the soothing, relaxed sensations that steal over them. When you go through your tension-release exercises, get in the habit of noticing how these two sensations feel in each part of your body: the hard, knotty feel and tug of the tense muscles; and the soothing, relaxing surge you feel once the muscles are slack.

The procedure at each stage of the exercise is always the same; tense the muscle as hard as you can, hold it for a slow count of five, and then relax it suddenly. Savor the pleasure that comes with the release for about fifteen seconds and tense the muscle one more time. Then move on to the next set. Each time you release a muscle, repeat to yourself the word *calm* or *peace* or *warm* or any similar word you think is appropriate. Now you're ready to start.

1. *Arms.* Start with whichever hand you favor. Clench it tightly, count, release, and enjoy the sensation. Do it twice. Now crook your arm and tense your bicep hard, following the same procedure. When that's done, repeat the process on the other hand and arm. Relax.

2. *Head and face.* First, raise your eyebrows as high as you can. Hold it. Release. Enjoy the sensation of the muscle release as it washes down over your forehead. Second, squint your eyes and wrinkle your nose hard, then release. Pause. Third, make the most exaggerated, forced smile you can. You should really feel the tension in your neck and jaw muscles. Relax. Pause.

3. *Neck and shoulders.* Drop your chin toward your chest but don't let it quite touch. Instead use your neck muscle to hold it back as though you were trying to prevent your chin from making contact. Concentrate on the tension, and the following release of the front neck muscles. Release. Relax. Now tilt your head back, using the same restraining technique to keep the back of your head from touching your shoulders. Your neck may shake slightly with the tension. Release. Relax.

Shift your attention to your shoulders. Spread them back as far as you can, until you feel the pull across the front of your chest. Release. Pause. Fold them forward, as though you were trying to touch them together in front of you. You should feel the tug across your back. Let them spring back. Relax. The last part of the shoulder series is an exaggerated shrug with your shoulders jammed up as high as you can put them. Let your arms hang loose so no excess muscle tension creeps into them. Hold. Release. Relax.

4. *Chest and stomach.* Take your deepest breath, hold for five seconds, and then release it s-l-o-w-l-y. Savor the calm that follows this. Pull in your stomach as far as you can when you inhale in this exercise, then let it settle out to its natural position.

5. *Buttocks, legs, and feet.* Make your buttocks as tense as you can, almost as though you're trying to raise yourself off the bed or chair by the effort. Count to five. Release. The release should bring a surge of relief through your lower back area. Next do your thighs, starting first on your favorite side and then doing the other. Tense. Relax each thigh. Once the thighs are relaxed, shift down to your calves. These muscles tend to cramp, so be a little more gentle when you tense. To tighten them, point your toes down and do your regular tense-relax ritual. Pause. When that is done, tense them again, this time pointing your toes up and back toward your face. Relax. As you do each of these exercises, study the tension first on the front of the foot and also on the front of your leg. You'll notice it doesn't take much to create it. The feet also have two tension exercises, pointing them out *à la* Charlie Chaplin, then relaxing; and later pointing them toward each other in a pigeon-toed pose. Do each series twice and notice how truly relaxed your feet will feel.

This is the whole body series. Depending on how proficient you become, it should take you between twenty minutes and a half-hour to do it all. Don't expect miracles at first. They will give you a mildly relaxed feeling the first few times. With practice and daily use the relaxing effects will build, so that before long you can produce soothing sensations to help you get to sleep with little effort. In the beginning at least, make an effort to practice the procedure twice daily if you can find the time. Make it a part of your day, like your coffee break or lunch hour, and schedule it for a certain time so you don't succumb to the "well, maybe tomorrow" syndrome. When you do it in the daytime, isolate yourself from any and all distractions, and once a session is over, enjoy that warm, relaxed feeling for a minute or two before you jump up and continue your day.

As you become more proficient you might want to increase the tension part of each tension-release cycle to about ten seconds, making sure always to keep repeating your relaxing word of *calm, warm,* or whatever you chose, as you release the tightened muscle. Some people find it helpful to be guided through these exercises by another soothing voice. If you feel you need that kind of reinforcement, you can get a prerecorded progressive relaxation instruction cassette through a service offered by *Psychology Today* magazine. Write: Psychology Today Cassettes, Dept. T48, P.O. Box 278, Pratt Station, Brooklyn, NY 11205; ask for cassette number 43, "Deep Relaxation." (At this writing, the price is $8.95; $9.95 if you are ordering outside the United States.)

Not everyone has the patience for all the counting, tensing, relaxing, and concentrating involved in the Progressive Relaxation process. All you may want at bedtime is something that will shake your body loose a little and work free some of those knots. Maybe all you need is a yoga exercise, not the kind where you do an imitation of a pretzel with your arms and legs, but a few simple exercises and postures that help you peacefully unravel.

The simplest of these is called deep breathing or the Complete Breath. You can do it as you're lying on your back in bed. It's a system of belly breathing that makes you feel as though you are purifying your lungs with new, clean air. First, lay your hands across your stomach, fingertips touching, just below your navel. Inhale, through the nose only, making the biggest belly you can. Slowly count to five as you do this. You should feel as though you are inflating yourself, filling your lungs to their capacity. Now exhale, again through the nose and again for a slow count of five. Feel the bubble of your stomach slowly decompress. Follow the easy, quiet rhythm of your breaths. If you do this breathing cycle fifteen or twenty times, before you finish you may find your eyelids slowly slipping down over your eyes.

A variation of this is something called alternate nostril breathing, which, as its name suggests, is simply breathing through one side of your nose at a time. The procedure is simple. Put the tip of the index finger of your right hand (or left hand, if you're left-handed) on your forehead and let your thumb and ring finger fall naturally to either side of your nose. (Again, this is strictly nose breathing, so you'll have to close your mouth.) Pinch shut your left nostril and leave your *right* one open. Inhale for a very slow count of five. Pinch both nostrils shut and hold the breath for another slow five count; then open your *left* nostril and let the air slowly move out for a last count of five. (As in the deep breathing exercises, make your belly do most of the work.) Try ten of these in-one-nostril-and-out-the-other cycles.

If you're looking for something just a little more strenuous, some type of mild exercise you can do before bed, you might try the pose known simply as the Cobra. You can do it in bed or on the floor in the next room if your bedmate objects. Lie on your stomach, legs together, feet stretched out, your hands palms-down on the floor near your head. Take five or six deep breaths. Give your body a little time to loosen up, then rest your forehead on the floor. Slowly raise your head up, inhaling as you move. Continue raising first your head and chin, then your chest, letting your lower back do some of the work. Then, using your arms in a kind of modified push-up, continue raising the upper part of your body off the floor. Everything from your waist on down should stay in contact with the floor during the whole exercise. Try to hold this posture for about ten seconds, or as long as it feels reasonably comfortable. Then slowly lower yourself down, exhaling as you go. Do this three times, *very* slowly. The point of the exercise is to relieve tension, not create it, so take it very easy.

When it's time to sleep, try the Savasana position, or pose of Complete Rest. It's not complicated—just lie on your back, with your arms lying limply by your side, palms up. Send your mind traveling through your body, starting with your feet, and gradually will your body to relax, one part at a time. Move up slowly from your feet to your calves, thighs, buttocks, the small of your back, abdomen, chest, shoulders, arms and down to your hands. Tense and release those muscles that are stubborn. Relax your face by letting your jaw go slack. If you have trouble keeping it loose, try "floating" your tongue inside your mouth so that it doesn't touch your palate or teeth. In time, you will feel your jaw slowly unclench. Think of your whole body as getting heavier, as though it's slowly sinking into the mattress.

While you're lying there, pay attention to your breathing. If you wish, you can practice your deep breathing at this time or just let your breath follow its own rhythm. Start counting breaths for as long as you want. (Do it at least until you hit twenty.) When you get bored with that, simply lie there and follow them. You'll find their steady metronome beat has a soothing effect.

All of these are *body* exercises—tinkering with your breathing and muscles to get your mind to unclamp its high-stress grip on you. The advantage of these exercises is that they are simple to learn, don't require the coordination and agility of a gymnast, and they are not tremendously taxing on the brain. The problem is, they sometimes don't work because they leave the brain alone. They give your mind time to rummage through the day's events and bother you with distracting thoughts while you're trying to get your Cobra pose down right or can't remember what you're supposed to tense next.

You can get around this either by giving your mind as much freedom as it can stand and letting it burn itself out; or you can make it work at putting you in the mood for a night's rest.

One of the let-the-thoughts-fall-where-they-may exercises is a technique developed by Harvard Medical School cardiologist Dr. Herbert Benson. He calls it the Relaxation Response, essentially a secular, scientific copy of transcendental meditation (TM®).

After studying the hypnotic, relaxing effects of the transcendental meditation technique and similar religious rituals that are soothing, Benson found they all had four main ingredients in common: a quiet environment; a verbal device, a word to act as a kind of white noise for the brain; a passive attitude; and a comfortable position. His main interest in studying them was as a cardiologist. He wanted to help people lower their blood pressure without depending so heavily on drugs. After testing his relaxation technique out on people, he found that it did that, and more. Those who faithfully followed the relaxation response found they were spontaneously cutting back on their intake of cigarettes, alcohol, and various legal and illegal drugs, as well as dropping their blood pressure. Benson was so impressed with the results he even suggested that businesses encourage their employees to take advantage of relaxation response breaks to help defuse some of the day's tensions and stress and to increase productivity.

It can also be a valuable sleeping pill but, like the progressive relaxation technique, it takes a little practice to get it up to full potential. Dr. Benson's prescription for his method is to do it twice daily: once in the morning or the middle of the day; and once before bedtime, for about twenty minutes each time. You can practice it almost anywhere, but ideally you should have a quiet room that is as free of distractions as possible. If you're worried about time, you can peek at your watch, but usually your own internal clock will work fine. The only thing you need is a comfortable chair. Now you're ready.

• Settle down in the chair, loosen your clothes, take your shoes off, get comfortable. Close your eyes.

• Take three or four deep yogic belly breaths and begin a relaxation survey of your body. From your toes up, start traveling through your body—feet, calves, lower torso, chest, shoulders, neck, and face—relaxing every muscle you can find. If one or two seem to fight you, try a little tense-and-release progressive relaxation to subdue it.

• Close your mouth and breathe only through your nose. Follow your breath. Every time you exhale, say the word *one* to yourself. If that word doesn't appeal to you, try another that does. How about *fun*? Or *money*? Or the traditional chant of meditators, *Om*? Whatever it is, it should have a soft, humming sound to it, one that will have a hypnotic effect when you repeat it over and over as you exhale. Typical in-out breath cycles would run: in . . . ONE, in . . . ONE, in . . . ONE; or in . . . MONNNEY, in . . . MONNNEY, in . . . MONNNEY.

• Do this for twenty minutes. (You can take a peek at your watch every now and then to see how much time has passed, but Benson advises against using a timer or alarm clock.) When the twenty minutes are up, sit quietly for a while, first with your eyes closed, then with them open.

And that's all there is to it.

You may be wondering how a normal, healthy human being can sit in one spot for twenty minutes, saying one word over and over again without getting a little restless or at least distracted by his or her own thoughts. This will happen, but as long as you're faithful to the basic formula, what Benson describes as a "wakeful hyometabolic," or very relaxed, state will assert itself. The key is that sound you're repeating to yourself. It can wash out just about any stray thought or concern with amazingly little difficulty. It's very much like the effect a group of chanting protesters get when they manage to drown out the words of a speaker and drive him from the podium. If you seem to have an unusually persistent thought, just have faith in your word repetition. It will jam all your stray thought waves if you let it.

The other bits of advice Benson offers, aside from practicing twice a day, is not to do this within two hours of eating a heavy meal, since the process of digesting your food seems to interfere with the technique. You may also feel a tingling in your body when you do relax. This is nothing to worry about. It is a very common symptom associated with the process. Finally, there is no way to "rate" each relaxation session. Every session will do you some good. Just let the relaxation occur at its own pace and forget about everything else. If, as you begin, you feel that twenty minutes is more time than you want to spend repeating one word over and over, try ten-minute sessions and work your way up to the twenty-minute level. The important thing is to do it faithfully twice each day, in the morning or early afternoon, and again in the evening, just before bedtime.

The relaxation response practically always works when taken as directed. The one big drawback in using it is that it has to be taken so often. Although you may have forty minutes each day to spare for sitting quietly in a room and buzzing out your stray thoughts, you also may not want to bother, especially if your insomnia is a sometime thing. Those who think they have a sophisticated level of self-control might want to try another technique by which their brains step in and trick the body into going to sleep. It's called Autogenic Training and was developed shortly after the turn of the century by a German neurophysicist, Dr. J. H. Schultz. He uncovered it while experimenting with hypnotism. He noticed that everyone who was hypnotized experienced two common sensations: their limbs always felt very warm and very heavy. Accordingly, he developed a series of suggestions that people could repeat to themselves and that would give the same effect of the hypnosis. They would say things like "My right arm is warm and heavy . . . warm and heavy . . . warm and heavy." And before they knew it, it would be. The process continues over the whole body, going from your arms to your head, shoulders, stomach, legs, and feet, each time with the hypnotic refrain, "My _____ is getting warm and heavy, warm and heavy." You can try it with the words, or try a slightly simpler variation, to imagine these sensations of heat and warmth oozing through your body. The advantages of this method are that it is completely silent; it involves no humming or thrashing around; and you can do it while you're lying in bed without disturbing the person sleeping next to you.

First you have to loosen up a little. Take about three deep yogic breaths and pick a spot on the ceiling to study; or project any image you feel like to fix on—a glowing red dot, a full moon, the pizza you had for lunch. The simpler the object the better. Fix your eyes on it and, while you study it, start counting your breaths every time you exhale. By the time you get to twenty, your eyelids should close by themselves. In spite of this, don't lose sight of your target; keep it fixed in your mind's eye.

Now think of warmth. The kind of slow, gentle heat that seeps into muscle and bone when you soak peacefully in a tub or stretch out languorously on a beach blanket under a July sun. Feel it move into your body, starting with your right arm. Notice how warm it is getting. How relaxed. You can barely move it. Feel your arm slowly settle into the mattress by your side. Now notice the same change coming over your left arm as well: the warmth, the relaxation, the sensation of it getting increasingly heavier. By now both your arms have become warm, relaxed, dead weight.

Shift your attention momentarily from your arms to your head and feel how that same wave of heat is slowly washing down from the top of your head and down over your forehead, eyes, cheeks, mouth, and down into your neck. Your neck is completely relaxed and your head is so heavy you can barely move it. It seems to be sinking more deeply into your pillow.

Gradually, this wave of warmth and relaxation will move down the length of your body. Feel the heat and trace its slow, deliberate movement down the back of your neck and into your shoulders. They are becoming warmer, more relaxed, heavier.

Follow the heat and relaxation as it travels down your spine into your lower back, your buttocks, and further down through your stomach. Let it trickle slowly into each leg, all the way down to the tips of your toes. Take your time as you feel it move. You're not going anywhere. Don't try to rush this natural relaxation process. It will proceed at its own rate. Wherever it arrives in your body, concentrate on the feeling of warmth, the way that part of the body gradually, almost imperceptibly, becomes heavier and more relaxed. By the time the process is finished, you will have a genuine sense of your body settling more deeply into the bed, as though it actually has gained weight and density. You feel warm and languid.

By this point, you may or may not be asleep. If you aren't, don't worry. You are so relaxed that sleep really isn't that far off. At this time start saying to yourself, "Waking does not matter, warmth makes me sleepy," over and over again in a slow deliberate way; or you can move on to the next step in using your brain as your sleeping pill.

First you have to do a little preparation. Start rummaging through your memory for a time or times when you felt completely relaxed and serene. It could have been a picnic on a warm spring day, paddling a canoe by yourself across a glassy smooth lake, or stretched out in front of a fire on a snowy winter night. Whatever they were, pick out your favorites and concentrate on what made them so special, so calm. Try to recall everything you can about them: the colors, the smells, the textures of things, that special feeling of serenity you had.

If you can't think of anything, fly a kite. Create a beautiful, breezy summer day for yourself, no clouds and all the room in the world to run. Pick up your kite, unroll a few feet of string and give it a tug to feed it to the wind blowing at your back. Watch it start climbing and feel it pulling on you, demanding more string. Little by little unreel your spool and watch the red (or any color you want) diamond shape rise into a crystal blue sky. Let your eyes follow the long, sweeping curve of string disappearing up toward that red spot climbing and diving in the air above you. Stretch out on the sun-warmed ground and watch your kite do its slow lazy dance at the end of the string. The breeze carries the smell of freshly cut grass to you. The summer sun feels warm and relaxing. You feed out more string and your kite is getting smaller and smaller and smaller. . . .

The important thing is to project yourself into any relaxing situation as totally as possible, trying to recapture as much of the change and movement around you, as well as all the sensations that came with the experience. It can be as complicated or as simple a scene as you want. (Some yogis suggest to their students that they imagine a perfectly calm pond between their eyes.) The only thing that counts is that it comes close to duplicating that original peaceful feeling.

It is possible to get the same sleep-inducing effect with a little reverse psychology. Psychologist Dr. Anees Sheikh of Marquette University has a technique he calls Eidetic Imagery. Very simply, it involves thinking of a time when you were miserable because you couldn't sleep, not because you didn't want to, but because some type of job or project was keeping you up working all night. You forced yourself to stay up studying for a big exam, or tying up the loose ends on a big project. Maybe you were just caught in the crunch of jet lag and had to fight off sleep long enough to get to your hotel.

Dr. Sheikh suggests you do the same memory projection as before, putting yourself back in that situation, feeling the fatigue, the aching hunger for sleep, the constant battle to stay alert. Take yourself up to what you remember as being the most wearing part of the night and, instead of going ahead and finishing whatever the job was, quit. Sheikh says at this point, when you should be drowsy from thinking about that experience, what you should do is say to yourself "Forget it. I'm not going to take the exam" (or whatever it was that kept you awake). If you did a convincing job of projecting yourself into that situation, you may find that the sleep you missed that night is going to come tonight. There is some justice in this world after all.

For a lucky few, all these relaxation tactics work without fail. A few deep yogic breaths or some quick muscle tensing and these fortunate ones are sound asleep. For most of us, however, insomnia isn't that easy to beat. We have to try a scattershot approach and hope that something blows it away. What you can do if you are up against the occasionally stubborn insomnia is try a kind of combination method, using a little of each of the techniques already outlined in this chapter. When you're finished, you may be sleeping. The strategy is simple: start from the outside and work in.

THE BODY

Begin by taking three deep yogic breaths to get you in the mood to relax. Remember to breath from your stomach and do it slowly for the count of five each time you inhale and exhale. Follow your breaths for a count of twenty as you fix your eyes on some object, real or imaginary, and close your eyelids if they haven't already closed.

Give yourself an Autogenic Therapy warm-up, letting that wave of heat seep through your body. Feel it spread up your arms to your head and back down through your neck, shoulders, stomach, back, buttocks, and legs. Everywhere it goes, feel the sensations of warmth and heaviness that it brings, weighing down your body with gradually relaxing muscles and limbs.

Lie there enjoying the warmth as you get ready to move on to the next step, a condensed version of Progressive Relaxation. It's not as elaborate, since it doesn't take each muscle separately, but it does follow the same general ritual. You will again tense the muscles for a slow count of five and release them suddenly to enjoy the calm that comes with the release. Take fifteen or twenty seconds to enjoy the sensation of the release of tension before moving on to the next muscle group.

Start with your upper torso. You're going to want to tense as much of your upper body as you can all at once. It's a simple procedure. Start by making two fists and squeeze. Feel the muscles knot up in your forearms and a little bit in your upper arms. Keep the muscle tension moving up your arms through your biceps and shoulders, across your chest and back. When everything is taut, hold it for five seconds, or as long as you can if that is too much, and then release all at once. Relax.

Next comes your face. Squint your eyes and wrinkle your nose. Hard. Hold this for about five seconds, and relax. Next wrinkle your brow and pucker your lips as though you are about to deliver a kiss that could kill. Pucker and hold it for a count of five, then relax. Finally, make the biggest, phoniest smile you can muster and stretch it one step beyond into an enormous grimace. Hold it for the five count and then relax.

Inhale. Try to touch your spine with your stomach. Push it in as far as you can and hold it there for the five count. Relax.

Lastly, curl your toes and, from your feet up, tighten gradually the lower part of your body, tightening your calves, thighs, and buttocks in one great smooth swoop of tension. Hold it. Then release it quickly. Enjoy that loose, unraveled feeling that comes deliciously over your body.

Lie there for twenty seconds or so and enjoy it.

THE MIND

There you lie. Calm. Soothed. Relaxed. And awake. Now it's time to do some traveling. Create an escalator in your mind or, if you wish, a glass-walled elevator. Now get on it. This is going to pass by ten floors, but it is a nonstop escalator. You won't have to get off until you reach the bottom.

There's really nothing to see. Just large blue numbers that move slowly by your eyes as you descend. You can take as much time as you want moving down past each level, the slower the better. As you pass each number on your smooth, floating descent, repeat it softly to yourself. "10 . . . 9 . . . 8 . . . 7 . . ." and so forth.

Once you reach bottom, what you'll find is one of your favorite peaceful settings from the past. A calm lake with the morning mist still curling off its surface, or a wide-open field of wildflowers that stretches on forever. A butterfly drifts through the air in front of you. You lay down in the tall, cool grass and watch its random movement from flower to flower. . . .

It doesn't necessarily have to be such a totally calm scene that you envision. I have one friend who enjoys (if that's the word) skydiving. When he wants to pull a relaxing memory out of his head, he makes a mental parachute jump.

"I think back on the peaceful part of the jump, after I've left the plane. There's a kind of floating sensation once you're out in the air there. You look at the plane and you don't feel like you're falling, but that the plane is slowly drifting up and away from you. I lie there, watch it for a while, and float along, the air brushing past my face," he recalls. "Then, when I pull the ripcord, there's instant silence. There's no quiet like it. Maybe the only noise I'll hear is the faint drone of the airplane somewhere above me, but that's it. On a bright sunny day the view is spectacular. I feel like I have all the time in the world to just sit there stuck up in the sky in complete peace and look around me. I enjoy the sun. I enjoy the view. I never feel like I'm descending but that the earth is gradually floating up toward me. I look down, pick out my landing spot, and pull on my control lines to aim me in the right direction. The earth is slowly moving up closer and closer. To land right I have to relax, bend my knees. I pick a huge pit filled with a lot of loose, white sand as my landing spot. It drifts up to me slowly. My feet touch ground. I fall gently over on my side with a soft thump. By the time I touch ground, I'm usually asleep."

This whole body-mind procedure is much less complicated than it sounds. The simplest way to remember it is as a four-part formula:

• Get comfortable. Perhaps try the pose of Complete Rest. Do deep yoga breathing to help you settle down.

• Take your body through a slow, body-warming session of Autogenic Therapy. Lie there quietly when it's finished.

• Now do the condensed version of Progressive Relaxation, tensing and relaxing first your upper torso, your head, your face, and finally your lower torso.

• Take your imaginary escalator ride for a slow count from ten down to one, till you arrive in one of your favorite peaceful scenes. Stay there as long as you want. Shift scenes if you get bored.

This exercise series will take a little while to complete—close to an hour if you do it properly. But if you can't sleep, time should be the least of your problems. There is no guarantee that this method, or for that matter any of the techniques described in this chapter, will work; but considering the alternative you have, any of these techniques is worth trying. You already know that if you simply lie there and worry, your insomnia is guaranteed, so anything else you try is bound to be more productive.

The best way to use all these relaxation techniques is on a daily basis, at least as part of your bedtime ritual. Most of the relaxation-method gurus recommend practice at least twice a day, for about twenty minutes a session. This is good advice, because all the techniques involve using body and mind skills that improve with practice. If you save them only for the occasional emergency, you won't be getting the full benefit. But you may not want to spend forty minutes per day on any of these methods. If that's the case, at least set aside ten minutes for one practice session before you go to bed. On good nights, this habit will get you to sleep faster. On bad nights, it will increase the odds of your getting any sleep.

There is one other method that, strictly speaking, doesn't really belong in this chapter. Everything that's been described entails exercise for the solo insomniacs who are left to fight their body tension on their own. If you have a kind and understanding bedmate who is willing to give about ten or fifteen minutes of his or her time before you go to bed, try a little massage. It doesn't have to be elaborate, just one or two exercises to help relax those tense muscles in the neck or back. While there are techniques of self-massage, most people don't find them very satisfying. Trying to massage yourself to relax is a little like tickling yourself to get a laugh. It's always better when someone else does it.

Massage works best when you're lying on a firm, padded surface, such as a carpeted floor, but you can do it in bed. You won't lose that much of the relaxing effect by doing it there, and you can go right to sleep when it's over. When you or your partner massage, use firm, even strokes and adjust pressure to the "massagee's" comfort level. This is not supposed to be a painful process, so be gentle and, of course, don't rub where there are bruises or injuries or joint or muscle problems.

There are whole massage rituals you can follow, but, as a presleep relaxer, one of these two might work. The first is for the neck. Let's assume for instruction's sake that you will be the one giving the massage. Have the person lie on his or her back and take three or four deep relaxing breaths. Kneel near the top of the person's head and, palms facing each other and fingers held together, reach down and cup the back of the neck in your hands. Lift the neck up slightly and start moving your hands like pistons, making slow, circular, up-and-down rubbing motions, a little like the movement your feet make when they're pedalling a bicycle. Press into the neck muscle gently on each upstroke. Practice will improve your touch and tell you how long you need to do it. Two or three minutes may be enough to start.

For the second exercise, have the person roll over on his or her stomach. Straddle the body so you are facing the head. Starting at the small of the back, place the heel of each hand on either side of the spine. Press down (the person on the bed will tell you how hard) rocking forward as you do. Rock back, lift your hands, and position them further up the spine. Now rock forward slowly, pressing firmly but gently, following the groove on either side of the spinal column. Go all the way to the top, the base of the neck, and then come back down in the same smooth, even, rocking motions. As a variation on this you might want to use your finger tips (index finger and ring finger) of either hand instead of the heels. You can get the same soothing effect by using much less pressure. Do this up-and-down run five to ten times, or until you can feel the back muscles relax.

These massage techniques should help get at some of that tension collected in those muscles at the base of your neck or in the small of your back. (If the idea of a more elaborate massage regimen appeals to you, a good how-to book on the subject is *The Art of Sensual Massage*, by Gordon Inkeles and Murray Todris, Straight Arrow Books.) These may not get you to sleep, but all that body touching might lead to some lovemaking. And that might be just what you need.

With your best efforts the worst can and often does happen. You may exhaust your repertoire of gimmicks and still be wide awake. Like it or not, you've suddenly been handed a gift of extra time. The best thing you can do is forget about insomnia, get out of bed, and make the most of it.

7.
The Compleat Insomniac

Maybe sometime in the future, around the year 2,000, say, twenty-first-century insomniacs will be able to stumble over to their push-button telephones in the middle of the night and tap out the toll-free, hot-line number 800-N-O-S-L-E-E-P for the national information network of Insomniacs Anonymous. In a matter of seconds, they can then find out what kind of late-night activities are on in their area that night, get a quick list of other insomniacs they can call to share their misery, or hear what the Sleep Suggestion for the day is. Restored with this information, they can then face the rest of the night as more serene individuals.

Unfortunately if you dial that number today you don't get very much, just a prerecorded voice coming out of the void of the phone system telling you to check your number, hang up, and dial again. It's a brutal fact of life that while people who are victims of everything from schizophrenia to hay fever have some group to turn to for help, the insomniac has to rough it alone.

Beyond a certain point, even the sleep experts are of little help. There are reams of reports and studies charting everything from the biochemistry and personality of insomniacs to their diet and daily habits. There are volumes written on ways to get to sleep as well, but once your battle for sleep is over, and you have lost, about the best advice you get from the experts is something like, "Don't worry about it. Tomorrow's another day." In the meantime, you're left with the rest of the night to kill.

When facing this situation, your best strategy is a good offense. Now that you have all this "found" time, you may as well enjoy it.

READING

The easiest place to start is with the solution everyone turns to in their sleepless misery, cracking open that book they've "always wanted to read." There are two schools of thought on insomniac reading: think dull; or think exciting.

The philosophy behind reading dull books is that you either get the chance to knock off a classic or maybe will get lucky and get a good night's sleep instead. If you're at a loss as to what to chose, you might want to start with the list of the 15 Most Boring Classics (see page 109) or, if you're looking for something a little more modern, how about James Joyce's *Finnegan's Wake*? (If you should actually read the whole thing, don't brag about it. No one will believe you.)

A corollary to the dull-book school of thought is the thick-book school. It's not that all long books are necessarily dull, it's just that, realistically speaking, when something starts slipping above the 300-page mark, you probably will find that your attention starts slipping with it. It could be a wav to get you back to sleep. A good thick-book selection could include:

Ulysses, by James Joyce
The Magic Mountain, by Thomas Mann
The Brothers Karamazov, by Fyodor Dostoyevsky
Practically anything by Charles Dickens
Anything by Alexander Solzhenitsyn

The exciting-book school of thought advises that as long as you're up, you may as well have a good time. What goes in this group will depend on your tastes. If you like nonsense and have a mind for brain games, for example, you might try *The Complete Works of Lewis Carroll* (Vintage Books). It has all the Lewis Carroll classics plus puzzles, games, problems, and acrostics devised by the mathematically minded author. Although it technically belongs on the thick-book list (it has 1,293 pages), it's more of a browser's book and a pleasant time-killer.

Many people find that mysteries suit those long nights perfectly, and we all have our favorite or favorites. Fortunately, the works of the best and most prolific mystery writers are all readily available in paperback, so they will be easy to find. If you have no preferences, or are looking for a starter set of the best of the mysteries, you might try:

The Big Sleep, by Raymond Chandler
The Murder of Roger Ackroyd, by Agatha Christie
The Hound of the Baskervilles, by Arthur Conan Doyle
The Maltese Falcon, by Dashiell Hammett
The Blue Hammer, by Ross Macdonald
The Five Red Herrings, by Dorothy Sayers

If you get hooked on any one of these writers, you're set for a good many nights. Every one of them has a lot more books ready to fill your late-night reading time.

For the person whose insomnia is more than a sometime thing, starting an insomniac bookshelf might not be a bad idea. Simply set aside a part of your bookcase for all those books—paperbacks you bought on impulse in airports, or the Solzhenitsyn books you bought out of guilt—that you never got around to reading. That way, as you come stumbling out of the bedroom you can head right for your shelf and have something there waiting.

MEET THE STARS

Astronomy is the perfect pastime for the insomniac who wants to get a little fresh air and something to look at. All you need is a guidebook for the stars (Try A *Field Guide to the Stars and Planets*, by Donald Menzel, Houghton Mifflin. It gives you a series of star maps that tell you what you see), two good eyes, and a clear night. (The last requirement may rule out this pastime for some smog-shrouded city-dwellers.) If you can get your hands on a pair of binoculars (eight power), so much the better.

There are over forty constellations you can spot with the naked eye. With binoculars, you can study pockmarks on the moon, see Jupiter and four of its twelve moons, and, looking closely, the rings of Saturn. If you get hooked on sky viewing, you will start developing an eye for seasonal shifts in the sky: night shows of comets and meteors, and meteor showers which appear on a predictable annual schedule. (The Perseids shower in mid-August is especially spectacular.)

It's a quiet, engrossing hobby that appeals to many night people (Johnny Carson among them). If you find yourself drawn to astronomy, you may want to get a telescope. You have a choice of three designs: the refractor type, the kind Galileo started out with; the reflector type, which uses a mirror and lens system; and exotic compound telescopes called catadioptrics, which are very sophisticated and expensive (over $3,000). Reflector telescopes give you the best combination of design and price. For a starter model, you should get nothing smaller than a six-inch reflector to enjoy star watching. Since it's an investment of a few hundred dollars for a good telescope, take the time to shop around before you plunge in and buy one. (Some experts feel one of the best choices available today is the Dynascope, made by Criterion Manufacturing Company, 620 Oakwood Avenue, West Hartford, CT 06110. Price: about $250.)

And, if you have any close encounters in the course of your sky viewing, the place to report them to is: Center for UFO Studies, 924 Chicago Avenue, Evanston, IL 60202.

PIECEWORK

For the woman or man who likes to work with his or her hands, there is the soothing and satisfying choice of putting together a patchwork quilt. The appeal of this pastime is that it is a totally involving process, putting not only your hands to work but your mind as well, as you arrange those kaleidoscopic designs with fabric swatches. There are no special artistic skills needed to start a quilt, and you can make one without any sewing background. All you need is time and an appreciation for design.

Quilting gives you a chance to create something of your own, learn a folk art, and have something to use in your bedroom on those chilly nights when you do sleep. Or you can display quilts on the wall as works of art (maybe on the wall facing the apartment of a noisy next-door neighbor).

Quilting is a hobby you can take your time doing (some of the old-time masterpieces took forty years) and one which will give you a real sense of satisfaction. Once you've tackled a quilt with the Martha Washington's Star design, for example, you can always move on to some pattern that is more challenging, such as Grandmother's Fan or Drunkard's Path. If you're interested in getting started, one of the best primers on the subject is called, logically, *The Perfect Patchwork Primer*, by Beth Gutcheon, Penguin Books.

If quilt making seems like too grand an undertaking, you can always try some other sewing or knitting activities. Stanford University sleep expert Dr. William Dement described one patient who could get only four hours' sleep per night and so spent much of his nighttime crocheting gifts for his friends. Others find tremendous relaxation in doing needlepoint, a pastime that football star Roosevelt Grier liberated for men to do as well as women.

LIFE BY THE NUMBERS

While you're sitting around wondering what's to become of you, you may as well take out your pocket calculator and figure it out in cold hard numbers. The first way is by a theory known as biorhythms. According to this belief, you are constantly going through three cycles of changes: a 23-day physical cycle; a 28-day emotional one; and a 33-day intellectual one. The first half of each of these cycles are all good days, so-called plus days, when you feel healthy, happy, and are sharp as a tack. You should do all your exercising, partying, and heavy thinking then. The second half of the cycles are all down days, negative days, when you're more inclined to feel tired, moody, and not too bright.

The real danger days are the halfway points in the cycles, known as the critical, or zero, days. That's when people are most likely to have accidents, get sick, or even die, because the body's system is out of balance. Custer supposedly made his famous blunder at Big Horn on a zero day, and the day of the battle at Waterloo was a zero day for Napoleon as well. If two biorhythms hit the critical mark on the same day (double zero) or if three do (triple zero), your chances of disaster are even greater.

Drawn out on a graph, these biorhythms look like sinuous up-and-down waves snaking above and below the critical zero line. If you want to go to the trouble, you can plot them out on a piece of graph paper, but a little addition and long division should be enough to give you an idea of where you stand.

The way you compute your biorhythms is simply to divide the total number of days you've lived so far by the three magic biorhythm numbers: 23, 28, and 33. (The theory says that every rhythm begins on the day you were born.) The remainders of this long division should tell you whether each cycle is in an up or down phase.

Let's take the example of a person who was born on March 8, 1936. On May 1, 1976, he decided to find out what his biorhythms were. The addition goes as follows:

Forty years of 365 days	14,600 days
Extra days for leap years	10 days
Days from March 8, 1976, to and including May 1, 1976	54 days
	14,664 days

Now we divide to find out what his biorhythms are doing.

• For the physical cycle: 14,664 ÷ 23 = 627 complete cycles and a remainder of 13 days.

• For the emotional cycle: 14,664 ÷ 28 = 523 completed cycles and a remainder of 20 days.

• For the intellectual cycle: 14,664 ÷ 33 = 444 completed cycles and a remainder of 12 days.

This shows that the person is heading into the bottom half of his twenty-three-day physical cycle and will probably be feeling a little sluggish for the next ten days. He is also twenty days into his emotional cycle, which means that during the next eight days, the low half of his cycle, he may feel somewhat depressed. Finally, he is still in the first half of his mental cycle and has a little over four good brain days ahead to get his heavy mental work done.

Another numbers game you might want to try to see what kind of year you've had is a special stress scorecard devised by psychiatrist Dr. Thomas Holmes to rate some of life's traumatic experiences. In testing it out, he found that 80 percent of the people who scored over 300 for a year's worth of these events suffered depression, heart attacks, or ulcers. Take a quick run through the list, make a tally of your life events, and add them up. Notice that both neutral (change in residence) and good (outstanding personal achievement) stresses can take their toll on you as well as the bad ones.

Life Event	Value
Death of a spouse	100
Divorce	73
Marital separation	65
Jail term	63
Death of a close family member	63
Personal injury or illness	53
Marriage	50
Fired at work	47
Marital reconciliation	45
Retirement	45
Change in health of family member	44
Pregnancy	40
Sex difficulties	39
Gain of new family member	39
Business readjustment	39
Change in financial state	38
Death of a close friend	37
Change to a different line of work	36
Change in number of arguments with spouse	35
Mortgage over $10,000	31
Foreclosure of mortgage or loan	30
Change in responsibilities at work	29
Son or daughter leaving home	29
Trouble with in-laws	29
Outstanding personal achievement	28

Life Event	Value
Wife begin or stop work	26
Begin or end school	26
Change in living conditions	25
Revision of personal habits	24
Trouble with boss	23
Change in work hours or conditions	20
Change in residence	20
Change in schools	20
Change in recreation	19
Change in church activities	19
Change in social activities	18
Mortgage or loan less than $10,000	17
Change in sleeping habits	16
Change in number of family get-togethers	15
Change in eating habits	15
Vacation	13
Christmas	12
Minor violation of the law	11

If you find you are veering close to the 300 mark, maybe it's time to slow down.

FAMILY, PAST AND FUTURE

Thanks to Alex Haley, there's a *Roots* mania in the United States. More and more people are taking a deeper interest in their past and are becoming avid family historians. If you've always had the urge to start digging, now may be as good a time as any. The basic equipment is simple: curiosity and a lot of time. All you need are a few key books and bits of information to steer you in the right direction.

The *Roots* craze has spawned a number of how-to books on doing a family history, but the best around is still *Searching for Your Ancestors*, by Gilbert H. Doane (Bantam Books), which is full of solid, commonsense advice. A good backup work on the topic is *The Genealogist's Encyclopedia*, by L. G. Pine (Collier Books), which gives advice on how to get at records of genealogical value in your ancestor's country of origin.

Start by finding out how much you know and don't know. Work up a skeleton chart, the kind where one line branches off into two lines, which branch off into four lines, and so on. It should read from left to right, starting with you, and branching off to your father's family, which traditionally runs across the top of the chart, and your mother's family, which runs across the bottom. Go back as far as you can to your grandparents and great-grandparents, leaving room to note when they were born, married, and died. (Don't clutter the chart with cousins, aunts, or uncles. All you want now is a strictly child-to-parent-to-grandparent flow that leads to you.)

Now get a loose-leaf notebook and allocate a page for each ancestral couple in your chart. On it note their full names, birthdates, birthplaces, marriage dates, dates of death, and places of burial. Finally, list the children—this is where your aunts and uncles come in—their dates of birth, marriage, and death, as well as birthplace. Once you've done all this, you should have a clear idea of what you need to find out.

Gilbert Doane's book will help you decide what to look for in local records, and you can also search the nation's gold mine of records, the National Archives, by mail. It's easy if you know how. While you have the time, start putting together a family historian's kit that will give you information about how to gain access to various government records.

For basic information on what's available in the National Archives, as well as in the record files of many state offices, write to:

Superintendent of Documents
U.S. Government Printing Office
Washington, D.C. 20402

and order the following books and booklets:

Guide to Genealogical Records in the National Archives, by Meredith B. Colket and Frank E. Bridgers; price, $1.65.

Where to Write for Birth and Death Records; price, $.35.

Where to Write for Marriage Records; price, $.35.

Where to Write for Divorce Records; price, $.35.

These will point you in the right direction for basic information sources. To get more specific information on the National Archives, write to:

National Archives and Records Service
General Services Administration
Washington, D.C. 20408

and ask for the following leaflets (they're all free):

Genealogical Records in the National Archives (General Information Booklet Number 5)

Military Service Records in the National Archives (General Information Booklet Number 7)

Location of Records and Fees for Reproduction Service in the National Archives (General Information Booklet Number 14)

Regional Branches of the National Archives (General Information Leaflet Number 22)

National Archives and Records Service Microfilm Publications (General Information Leaflet Number 24)

Federal Population Censuses, 1790–1890 (This is a catalogue of microfilm copies of old censuses that you can buy from the National Archives.)

With what's found in these publications, you can search practically any free-access system of records the government has, and, in many cases, do it all by mail. This opens up everything from old land records and censuses to military rosters and passenger lists which could help you fit together the missing pieces of your family puzzle. If you decide to start the project, keep your file of records on your insomnia shelf—that way you can work on it in the peace and quiet of one of those long nights.

If your family concerns are directed more to the future than the past (and if you are a woman), you could use your insomnia time to work up baby-sex prediction charts, so you know whether or not to paint that spare bedroom pink or blue.

Sex prediction techniques seem to have their fads, like everything else. Back in the 1960s, gynecologist Dr. Landrum Shettles developed what he claimed was a pick-a-boy/pick-a-girl system that was 85 percent accurate. In practice, it didn't seem to work that way. One gynecologist recommended the technique to his patients and the first thirty that tried it all got the exact opposite sex of what they wanted.

Shettles's method has since been eclipsed by a discovery made by Dr. Roderigo Guerrero at Harvard Medical School. In a statistical study of conception and birth, he discovered that women impregnated close to their ovulation time had a higher number of girls, while those who became pregnant a number of days before ovulation seemed to have more boys.

A colleague of his, Dr. Elizabeth Whelan, has translated Guerrero's findings into a system of sex selection which she says can tilt slightly the natural 51-49 boy-girl odds that nature gives you. Essentially, she claims that having sex on each of the two days prior to ovulation and on the day of ovulation itself will give you a 57 percent chance of having a girl. Intercourse on the sixth, fifth, and fourth days before ovulation will give you a 68 percent chance of having a boy. Slightly chauvinistic, I know, but that's the way it works.

What the woman must do is figure out in advance when her ovulation will be coming. She can do this by a simple morning routine of taking her temperature before she gets out of bed and noting the temperature immediately on a chart. The reason for this routine is that the woman's body temperature dips slightly, about four-tenths of a degree or so, one or two days before ovulation. Like the menstrual cycle, ovulation follows a regular schedule, so after taking and charting her morning temperature for two or three months, a woman should be able to predict, within a day or so, when her ovulation is due. (Most women find that it comes fourteen to fifteen days after menstruation.)

To do this, all you need is an oral thermometer and charts for each month. You can use graph paper or draw your own graph-paper design. On the left side of the graph, starting from the bottom and going up, let each horizontal line represent a .2-degree increment in temperature; so the chart would read, from bottom to top: 97.0, 97.2, 97.4, 97.6, 97.8, 98.0, 98.2, 98.4, 98.6, 98.8, 99.0, 99.2, 99.4, 99.6. Across the top let each vertical line represent a day of the month. Each morning when you get up, all you have to do is find the right temperature-day intersection on your graph and draw a line from the previous day's intersection to that day's intersection. After a few months of doing this, says Dr. Whelan, you should have a good idea of ovulation day and be ready to give this mildly Brave New World type of experiment the acid test.

PRAYER POWER

Stress expert Dr. Hans Selye points out that many of the "new" ways to relax are basically different versions of religious rituals which we have had for years as various forms of group prayer or litany. These new methods have basically rediscovered what most religious people already know, that prayer can be physically as well as spiritually soothing. One way you can take advantage of this effect is by taking out your copy of the Bible and reading through your favorite book or passages until some of the aggravation and worry of not being able to sleep recedes. If you don't have a favorite, try the Book of Job. As a piece of literature, it is beautifully crafted and richly poetic. As an insomniac reading selection, it offers special consolation, since Job was a fellow sufferer. "Like a slave who longs for the shadow, and like a hireling who looks for his wages, so I am allotted months of emptiness, and nights of misery are apportioned to me. When I lie down I say, 'When shall I arise?' But the night is long, and I am full of tossing till the dawn," he complains.

If you are a religious Catholic, and want to share the night with others, you may want to consider joining the Nocturnal Adoration Society. Its members spend an hour in nighttime private and silent prayer once a month in one of the 550 churches that are branches of the organization. Any Catholic can join; there are no dues and no obligations other than to show up for your one hour of monthly prayer, which is scheduled on a rotating system all through the night. The purpose of these nightly prayer gatherings is to pray for the world, which needs all the help it can get.

If you are interested in joining, write the national headquarters of the Nocturnal Adoration Society, 194 East 76th Street, New York, NY 10021. They will send you further information on the society and tell you where to find the society branch that is nearest to you.

THE INSOMNIAC AS IRATE CONSUMER
AND CITIZEN

Maybe you didn't show up on the now-famous enemies list of the Nixon administration, or you haven't been called yet by one of those junk-phone-call robots, but your paranoia has never been keener. You're convinced they're all out there waiting to get you. You want your privacy back.

Let's start with junk mail. One Portland, Oregon, man saved his year's worth of unsolicited mail and found he had been sent 1,094 separate pieces of mail, a total of 75 pounds of paper. If you want to save your mailman the trouble of hauling all that paper to your door, and save the garbage man the work of hauling it all away, you can write to junk mailers and ask them to pull your name from their list, or get a copy of Form 2150 from the Post Office and put on it the names of the firms you do not want to be sending you their literature. The form should ensure that the mail is pulled before it gets to your door.

An even simpler solution, according to *Consumer Reports*, is to write to: Direct Mail/Marketing Association, Inc., 6 East 43rd Street, New York, NY 10017. Ask for their Mail Preference Service form, fill it out, and return it. Roughly 400 direct mail outfits belong to this association and, as a group, they account for over 70 percent of the third-class consumer, or junk, mail that goes out every year. When the association receives your completed form, it will purge your name from all these lists.

For the ultimate in mail protection you can enlist the services of a firm that will intercept and handle your mail for you. There is a published list of these firms that costs $4.00. It's called the *Directory of Mail Drops in the U.S. and Canada*, and you can get it from: Loopmanics Unlimited, P.O. Box 264, Mason, MI 48854.

You may also fear that yours is one of the approximately 20 million names stored in one of the FBI's 1,976 record systems. Your key to finding out is the 1974 Freedom of Information Act. The only catch is, you have to know how to ask for the information. You can't just write to the FBI and say, "What have you got on me?" You have to have some idea of the kind of information the bureau might have. It could be anything from record of an arrest at an antiwar demonstration to having been checked for a government or government-related job that may have required a security clearance of some kind.

All you have to do is write to: U.S. Department of Justice, Federal Bureau of Investigation, Washington, D.C. 20535, and describe as specifically as you can the kind of information you want to check on. It could be your arrest record for that sit-in, the security investigation for the job, or possibly even an investigation into some organization you once joined. Give whatever details—dates, locations, employers, circumstances—that would help them track down the information, and, for legality's sake, the letter should begin: "Under the Freedom of Information Act, 5 U.S.C.552, I hereby request access to . . ." and put your description here. By law the agency has to respond within ten working days of receiving your request. They won't release any information without getting your signature, birthdate, social security number, and fingerprints. (They will supply you with a card for that.) Good luck.

THE SOCIAL INSOMNIAC

Take a bracing, cool shower, slip on your best party clothes, and go out dancing. If you've already reconciled yourself to staying up most of the night, you may as well have fun while you're doing it. There's a lot to be said for dancing. Psychologically, it gets you out of your self and keeps your mind off your insomnia and the depression that may come with it. It practically guarantees that you will get to sleep when you get back home, and, if you're looking for a healthy reason, it's good exercise. A fast dance burns up about seven calories per minute, about the same burn-up rate as bicycling at a brisk pace. If you don't want to dance, try the telephone. If you live in or near a city of any size, they probably have an all-night talk show on a local radio station. Tune them in and see what's going on. Everyone wants to be a talk show guest—maybe this is the night you make your debut. Don't feel shy. You're not alone. One all-night talk show in New York claims that between 8,000 and 10,000 calls regularly jam the station's switchboard each night.

Another thing to remember is that when it's night where you are, it's always day somewhere else. If you have a friend or relative in another time zone, give them a call. There's less competition for the phone lines, the night rates are cheaper, and besides, it's a good antidepression tactic.

THE INDUSTRIOUS INSOMNIAC

It's not the big things, it's the little things that get you down, like that growing mass of ice swallowing up everything in your freezer, the birthday card you bought but never mailed, that pile of magazines you haven't read yet, or all those thought-provoking articles and recipes you clipped out that are jammed into one big wad of paper in a drawer. They're all not important enough in themselves to make your life miserable, but, confronted at the wrong time, they become the straw that breaks the insomniac's back. If this is part of your problem, if it seems like the edges of your life are frayed and a little out of control, maybe you can gather up the loose ends with an insomniac's work file. It could be nothing more than a slip of paper with a list of all those things you meant to do but somehow never got around to finishing. As each sleepless night comes, pull out your list, do one of the items, check it off, and put the list away until the next night. Then you can file those recipes, or hack out your freezer, or read the magazines.

Some suggestions:

• *Organize* your vacation slides or family album. Check your medicine cabinet. Throw out all those dust-covered tubes, bottles, and containers of stale prescription drugs that are crowding everything off the shelf. Check if you have the following basics on hand: aspirin, rubbing alcohol, hydrogen peroxide, an antacid, an antidiarrhea medicine, calamine lotion, petroleum jelly, two thermometers (one rectal, one oral), a roll of two-inch bandages, sterile gauze squares (four-inch size), one roll of adhesive tape, and one first aid book (the National Red Cross's *Standard First Aid and Personal Safety* guide is a good choice. Your local chapter should have copies.) Write down what you don't have and buy it, tomorrow. Or get the needed items at an all-night drugstore tonight.

• *Revamp* your phone/address book, making especially sure you have listed in a convenient place numbers for: family doctor or doctors, dentist, ambulance service, the nearest all-night drugstore, the local Poison Control Center, as well as, of course, the police and fire department.

As long as you're looking in your book, update names and addresses of friends and business acquaintances and maybe take the opportunity to work up that Christmas card list you never have when you need it.

• *Plan* a new you. Rip everything out of your closets and put into a Salvation Army pile anything you haven't worn in the last two years. (There's probably a good reason for that.) Those see-through body shirts, your orange Bermuda shorts, the tie with the map of the Yucatan silkscreened on it. Dump them. See how much better you'll feel.

Plan a replacement wardrobe, a new hairdo, a *realistic* diet, or an exercise regimen that you think you can follow.

• *Do* something you've never done before. Try some Zen or yoga exercises, some meditation, take up needlepoint, read haiku poetry, or, better yet, try to write some—start a diary or journal. Follow your impulses and see where they lead you.

FOR THE TRAVELING INSOMNIAC

Ten places in which it's not so bad to be sleepless:

1. *Las Vegas.* A mecca for hyperactive night people. It's a nonstop city that is designed for those who think sunlight is a natural pollutant.

2. *New York City.* If you have the time (and the money), you will find it very easy to pass the time here until dawn.

3. *Paris.* Even more elegant at night. Take an early evening elevator ride up the Eiffel Tower and see for yourself.

4. *Rio de Janeiro.* "Once you've seen Rio, you can forgive God for having made New Jersey," quipped one Rio-phile. The best time for the insomniac to come is during Carnival, the four-day party preceding Lent.

5. *Baltimore.* Baltimore? Yes, because they are kind to insomniacs in Baltimore. If you're in the area and sleepless, call (301) 653-2998, for Rent-A-Tour, an agency that conducts an insomniac's tour of the city, complete with a reading of "Annabel Lee" at Edgar Allen Poe's grave.

6. *Taj Mahal.* A jewel of an architectural creation, this white alabaster mausoleum was built by the emperor of the Moguls, Shah

Jahan, for his beloved and favorite wife, Mumtaz Muhal, who died while giving birth. On everybody's list of the wonders of the world, it is best viewed in the silver light of a full moon.

7. *Mt. Kilimanjaro.* A four-day hike takes you up to the top of the 19,000-foot peak, the "roof of Africa," in Tanzania. The last day begins at one o'clock in the morning so you can reach the peak in time to see the sun rise over Africa from the highest point on the continent.

8. *The Ark.* A modern, all-night game-viewing lodge in Aberdare Park, Kenya, where the insomniac will be rewarded with the night's procession of elephants, antelope, hyenas, and others trotting to and from the lodge's water hole.

9. *Machu Picchu.* The famous ghost city in Peru, perched 9,000 feet up in the Andes, between the twin peaks of Huyana Picchu and Machu Picchu. The spectacular view of this stone city in the sky is further enhanced if you stay overnight at the Machu Picchu Hotel and watch the sunrise over the ruins.

10. *Mont St. Michel.* A magnificent pile of stone—a medieval town, ancient monastery, and magnificent church all crammed onto a large tooth of granite that forms an island off the west coast of France. The best way to enjoy it is to stay overnight on the island during the night of a full moon so you can see the spectacular sight of the tide rushing from nine miles out over the sand flats at speeds of up to 210 feet per minute.

AND FOR THE INSOMNIACS WHO THINK THEY HAVE EVERYTHING

1. *Home computers.* For about $2,000 you can get a typewriter-console home computer which you can program to do everything from balancing your checkbook to playing brain games with you on those long lonely nights. Processor Technology Corporation (7100 Industrial Drive, Pleasanton, CA 94566) has a home brain for you in the person of its star model, Sol System II.

2. *Videorecorders.* If there's nothing on television worth watching at two in the morning, you can do your own programing with a videorecording of your favorite old movie or TV special. Prices for this very expensive toy hover between $1,000 and $1,500, depending

on how good a shopper you are. Right now there are only three brands on the market for home use: the Sony Betamax, JVC Vidstar, and the RCA Selectavision. All give you the options of taping one program while watching another and taping programs when you're not at home. Large department stores are also starting to sell $50 video-cassettes of first-run movies to pop in your machine or, if that doesn't appeal to you, you can always spring for the optional television camera and create your own after-midnight show.

3. *Computer chess.* Chess fanciers can pit themselves against the microcircuits of the Chess Challenger, a $200 toy available in many department stores and from: Lectro-Media, Ltd., P.O. Box 1770, Philadelphia, PA 19105. Different programing packages can boost its chess IQ if you feel that the two of you are mismatched.

4. *Wenger Sound Module.* The perfect place to practice on your tuba or primal screaming at three o'clock in the morning, this is a "sound controlled," prefabricated, glass-walled room that you can set up anywhere. Sizes vary from thirty-nine square feet to a hundred square feet, and prices range from about $4,000 to well over $6,000. If peace and quiet mean that much to you, contact: Wenger Corporation, Owatonna, MN 55060.

THE FINAL SOLUTION:

If you really get restless, go out and join the night people. The next chapter will tell you how.

8.
Children of the Night

"They're like moles. You can spot them on the street, in the daytime, white pasty skin, dark, hollowed-out eyes, looking a little dazed."

"No normal person lives like that. They're all running away from something."

"I'd say they are probably loners or losers or both. They just don't want to be a part of the life the rest of us follow."

These are some of the results of a totally random, unfunded, and unscientific survey of typical attitudes toward that most shadowy of all individuals in society, the night person. It's hard to find anyone who will say anything complimentary about someone whose "day" begins when everyone else's is ending. You can do your own amateur psychoanalyzing about why people think this way: a basic fear of the dark, and people of the night; being brainwashed by all those vampire, werewolf, and Frankenstein movies in which coffins open, bandages come unraveled, and mild-mannered people become fanged monsters once the sun goes down; or just the basic assumption that anyone who chooses the darkest, coldest, most unfriendly part of the day as his or her natural environment cannot be normal. Whatever the reason, the status of anyone who follows the life of a night person is only slightly higher than Typhoid Mary's was at the height of the epidemic.

This is the kind of company insomnia puts you in. It's bad enough that you can't sleep, but the fact that you have automatically become a member of a silent minority of misfits and neurotics is doubly demoralizing.

The problem with these attitudes is that they are solidly based on unsound popular misconceptions. Common sense has such a monopoly of what we "know" about night people in general, and insomniacs in particular, that few people pay any attention to the established facts on the subject. Sleep experts are finding out that all those bits of common sense about the insomniac and the night person really don't make all that much sense after all.

Take the notion that all insomnia is unhealthy, for example. Sleep experts are pretty much agreed that we all need sleep. That is a safe enough conclusion. Going to sleep every night seems to come with having a healthy body and mind. Few people can go more than a day without getting at least a few hours sleep. Problems come when scientists have to explain *why* sleep is healthy.

So far they haven't been able to tell why. At the moment, the answer is a toss-up between the two main sleep theories: the restorative one, which states that sleep is repair time for the body and brain; and the adaptive behavior theory, which says that sleep is a body habit left over from Stone Age times when humans were better off unconscious at night than wandering through prehistoric swamps and jungles. Although, as you've seen, the restorative theory is the one that makes the most common sense, no one has been able to back it up with proof— which brings up another problem: since the experts can't tell us why we need sleep, they also cannot tell us why insomnia is so bad.

No one is certain about what insomnia does to us. The more evidence the experts gather, the more elusive the answer gets. In 1959, for example, a New York disc jockey named Peter Tripp announced that he would stay awake and keep broadcasting for eight days without sleep as part of a fund-raising, publicity gimmick for the March of Dimes. During his broadcast breaks, a team of psychiatrists, psychologists, and specialists of all kinds was on hand to examine him and to help him through the ordeal.

After the fourth day without sleep, strange things started happening. He began having hallucinations that continued off and on through the rest of his sleepless marathon. A clock on the wall began to take on the features of the face of Dracula; he was convinced he saw flames surging out of a bureau drawer in the hotel room where he was staying. He had especially bizarre hallucinations about the doctors and scientists examining him. One doctor's tweed suit turned into a mass of worms before his eyes. Another man's tie kept twitching and jumping about like a dying snake and, while being examined by a doctor on the last day of the broadcast, Tripp was convinced he had been asked to strip and lie on a table as part of preparations to bury him alive.

All these·delusions and visions evaporated after one long night's sleep of thirteen hours at the end of Tripp's ordeal, but the experts had seen enough to be convinced that losing sleep could do horrible things to a person's mind. It confirmed much of what they had suspected all along.

Then in 1964 a seventeen-year-old San Diego high-school student, Randy Gardner,·stayed awake for eleven days as part of his science fair project, and some of the same experts went to watch. He was a big disappointment. He didn't act crazy the way he was supposed to. There were no wormy suits, no flames, and no illusions of premature burials. The only thing that seemed to happen from being up all that time was that he became very, very tired. The experts were, and are, totally confused.

Even in tests where they have created insomniacs by keeping normal people awake and where they amassed a small mountain of information, they were able to draw few definite conclusions. In fact, after years of study, the experts have agreed on only one finding: ·"The effect of sleep deprivation," pronounces University of Florida's Dr. Wilse Webb, "is to make us sleepy."

While some scientists are trying to puzzle out what insomnia can do *to* us, others have been working on what it can do *for* us. "We don't know that insomnia is *always* bad for us," says Dr. Charles Pollok of Montefiore Hospital's Sleep-Wake Disorders Clinic in New York City. "In some cases it actually seems to help people—those who are depressed, for example."

Many sleep experts are now finding that insomnia can be powerful medicine against depression. Up in Canada, McGill University psychiatrist Dr. M. Cole has been treating seriously depressed elderly patients with carefully prescribed doses of enforced insomnia, known as sleep deprivation, since 1971. He got the idea after reading a report by a couple of Dutch doctors about how some of their chronically depressed patients had a home remedy for their black moods—staying up all night.

One patient, a teacher, said he routinely went for all-night bicycle rides whenever he felt depression creeping over him. By the following morning he found his mood had lifted and he was completely recovered. Another patient, himself a doctor, said he was able to keep his depression in check by working all though the night as often as every two or three nights a week. He not only managed to do huge amounts of work this way but was feeling better as well.

Inspired by this report, Dr. Cole adopted the insomnia method for treating some of the elderly patients he was seeing in a nearby mental hospital. He worked out an insomnia dose thirty-six hours long and, depending on how bad a patient's depression was, he would prescribe one or two doses per week until the depression cleared up. After just one session of a day and a half without sleep just about every patient felt a kind of a "high" from the effects of sleep deprivation, a high that lasted about a day.

You've probably felt this amphetaminelike kick after forcing yourself through some kind of all-night session. After a while you no longer feel sleepy, but may instead feel a little lightheaded and hyperactive as well. In trying sleep deprivation on a group of depressed patients at the National Institutes of Health, doctors there found that after one dose many of their patients acted alert, energetic, and, in some cases, genuinely giddy from the effects. Cole himself found that by adjusting the dose to his patients' depression, he could use this "up" effect of insomnia to punch through their gloom.

Some of the results he got were dazzling. Cole had one patient, a seventy-eight-year-old widow, who had been suffering spells of depression for almost thirty years. After just one thirty-six-hour spell without sleep her depression lifted, her appetite improved, and she stayed recovered for well over a month. Other depressions took a little longer to crack. There was another widow in the same hospital who had already been through three months of standard antidepression therapy with no progress. She was seventy-five years old and had had problems with her depression since the death of her husband. After one sleep deprivation session her depression broke. She became more outgoing, talkative, and began taking an interest in life once again, writing letters to friends and family. This lasted for about a day. Then she slipped back into her old lethargy. Each time she would slip, Cole would prescribe another thirty-six hours of no sleep. Finally, after twelve of these sessions, her depression was cured.

Over a six-year period, Cole says, he has managed to help three-fourths of the seriously depressed patients he treated this way, and he believes this kind of controlled insomnia makes an ideal antidepressant drug, especially since it has practically no side effects.

Other doctors agree and have achieved equally encouraging results by using sleep deprivation on depressed patients. A National Institutes of Health research team got temporary cures of depression in ten out of nineteen of their seriously depressed mental patients. In addition, they found that, with the insomnia treatments, the worse the depression the better the recovery.

Why should no sleep cheer up someone who's depressed? It seems that eliminating sleep to beat depression is like taking up smoking to cure lung cancer. The reason why this may work, according to Emory University psychiatrist Dr. Gerald Vogel, is because of a certain change that goes on in your brain when it shifts into your dreamy REM, or rapid-eye-movement, sleep. The process that set REM sleep in motion, says Vogel, can also produce a natural antidepressant for the body. By not allowing the body to go to sleep, he says, you stir up a genuine craving or hunger for REM sleep that he calls REM pressure. And as this pressure builds, so does the amount of natural antidepressant chemical seeping into your bloodstream.

Vogel got the idea for this theory after looking over the most effective therapies for depression. He noticed that the best techniques and drugs all had one odd thing in common: they wiped out a person's REM sleep. Conversely, he noticed that drugs that *increased* depression also increased REM sleep. Intrigued by these insights, Vogel decided to skip the antidepressant drug, and to remove the REM sleep himself and watch what happened. He did this simply by hooking up a depressed patient to a sleep monitoring machine; every time the person started to drift into REM sleep, Vogel would wake him up by softly calling out his name.

He soon found that his method worked and did best on those with endogenous depression, that devastating kind of depression that springs up for no apparent reason and is often serious enough to require hospitalization. It is usually longer lasting and more serious than the other depression, called reactive because it is triggered by a specific life crisis, such as divorce or the death of someone close.

On one test run using this technique alone, with no drugs, Vogel managed to wipe out the depression of half of one group of thirty-four mental patients. A typical case he handled was that of a forty-seven-year-old woman who was severely depressed and who had been hospitalized after she attempted suicide by slashing her wrists. Vogel took her off all drugs and put her through his special REM-less sleep treatment. After three weeks, she was recovered well enough to go home.

His treatment has proved so successful that others are adopting it to use alone and in combination with antidepressants to speed up the cure of depressed mental patients. This does not necessarily mean that you can make a depression disappear simply by staying up all night. It could mean, however, that on those nights when you are depressed, the reason you can't sleep is because your brain is trying to heal itself and right your psychological equilibrium.

Besides lifting your depression, insomnia may also put a little more zing in your sex drive, according to one study done at Stanford University. The study involved ten men, some of whom had their REM sleep blocked out during a night in the sleep laboratory. The following day, they were asked to sit in small, enclosed booths equipped with special cameras that could follow where their eyes looked.

The men were told they were taking a special test to study "pupillary response to varying thematic content" and that a series of pictures would be flashed in front of their eyes for them to look over. What they weren't told was that the lineup of pictures was deliberately salted with four reproductions of art that had "young, attractive human females in varying states of undress." They included famous works such as *Odalisque and Slave* by Ingres, and *Persephone* by Thomas Hart Benton. The result of this picture-watching exercise showed that those who had been robbed of REM sleep the night before were scanning the art reproductions more like *Playboy* centerfolds than art masterpieces. In the words of the study, with the REM-deprived crowd the "sexual areas of the picture were fixated more frequently." Those that had a whole night's sleep seemed to have a more general, aesthetic appreciation for the art and didn't linger on the pictures' erogenous zones.

The Stanford scientists couldn't really answer the obvious question of why losing this one part of sleep should act like an aphrodisiac. They did offer a couple of theories. One is that REM sleep helps strengthen that part of your psyche that is in charge of controlling your impulses, basic appetites, and urges that come leaking out of what Freud called your id, the nonrational, animal side of you. Without that one night of REM sleep, your impulse control could get sloppy and, before you know it, you're leering at every picture of a naked man or woman you see.

Another theory is that some of the effects of losing REM sleep are that a person becomes restless, almost hyperalert, and sometimes a little aggressive as well—all effects that would help a human or animal survive a little better by keeping him on his toes. It's possible that this sexy side to losing REM sleep promotes another kind of survival, the survival of the species, by stimulating what the sleep experts delicately describe as "mating behavior." So if you've ever felt the distinct need for some mating behavior after a sleepless night, now you know the reason.

Besides being generally unhealthy, insomnia—common sense has always told us—has a kind of dry-rot effect on our minds. You know the feeling the day after a bad night of sleep or a night without any sleep—that stupor, the way your body has turned to sludge, that invisible headband tightening around your head. You feel stunned. It's pure agony.

For this reason insomnia has the whiff of torture or brainwashing about it to many people. Certainly no one sees it as doing the brain any good. But, if you can believe it, insomnia can work *for* the brain as well as *against* it. Being without sleep does not necessarily mean being without a clear working mind. A little insomnia before a big mental task of some kind, such as taking a test or reading a mass of complicated business reports or technical papers, for example, can be to your benefit. A series of memorizing experiments done by psychologist Dr. Bruch Ekstrand at the University of Colorado turned up the fact that even a short nap before tackling a learning project can foul up the brain's memory mechanism. "The procrastinator's approach— sleep before you learn—won't help your memory at all," psychologist Eric Hoddes wrote on the study in *Psychology Today* magazine. "In fact, a short period of sleep just before new learning can seriously increase forgetting. . . ."

One reason for this memory block, says Hoddes could be a hormone called somatotrophin that is released during sleep. In experiments with animals he found that mice injected with this hormone before being taught how to run a maze had a harder time remembering how to do it again than those mice that got their injections after maze training. If this works the same way in people, Hoddes says, then you're better off getting no sleep at all before you put your mind to work.

That insomnia which is driving you crazy may also give your memory a little boost. One University of California experiment took two groups of people and gave each a word list to look over. One group was then told to go on with their normal day, while the other was told not to sleep that night. The following morning, both groups took memory tests to see how well the words stuck. The insomniacs beat the sleepers hands down, showing the best recall of what was on the list. So it looks like insomnia not only gives you the time to learn something but also gives you the brainpower to remember it as well.

As a brain-aid, insomnia does not get very much publicity. (Most of the attention and publicity concentrated on it is geared to wiping it out, a miracle which, judging by the body count of between 20 and 35 million insomniacs, medicine is not pulling off very well.) As an example, all the credit for anything creative that happens at night usually goes to dreams. Pick up any sleep or dream book and you'll read about how Samuel Taylor Coleridge wrote *Kubla Khan* after seeing the whole poem in a dream, or how Robert Louis Stevenson got his inspiration for *Dr. Jekyll and Mr. Hyde* from a dream, or how German scientist Frederick August Kekule made his discovery of the structure of the benzene molecule after seeing six snakes form a hexagon shape in a dream.

But you never read about the creative contributions that insomnia makes. Granted, inspirations are usually hard to come by when it's 3:00 A.M. and you can barely focus your eyes. Most often you are not thinking about writing the Great American Novel or coming up with a million-dollar idea. There are people whose creative flow seems to thrive on insomnia or, at least, very little sleep. One of the best known was the writer Franz Kafka. His diaries are full of entries such as "Slept, awoke, slept, awoke, miserable life," and "Let me only have rest at night—childish complaint," which documented a lifelong familiarity with insomnia.

Unlike most people, Kafka didn't see his sleeplessness as a curse so much as a hopeful sign that ideas which had been brewing inside were ready to come to the surface and be written down. "I believe this sleeplessness comes only because I write," he entered in his diary in 1911. And a few years later: "If I can't pursue the stories through the nights, they break away and disappear. . . ." He had a kind of love-hate relationship with insomnia which gave him both the opportunity and impetus to write.

Another person who welcomed as little sleep as possible was Thomas Alva Edison. A strong-willed, high-energy individual, he was always fighting to beat back sleep so he would have time to work on his many creative projects. He usually tried to keep his sleep down to four or five hours at night and took short naps during the day to keep going. He had practically no use for the standard eight-hour dose of sleep that everyone was supposed to get. In what is probably his most famous pronouncement on the subject, he wrote, "Most people overeat one hundred percent and oversleep one hundred percent. . . . That extra hundred percent makes them unhealthy and inefficient." He was hoping that his light bulb would help people trim off that excess hundred percent.

Others simply prefer to take advantage of what time insomnia gives them. "If you don't fight against those sleepless nights," says Dartmouth sleep expert Dr. Peter Hauri, "you can enjoy them. Usually I find I can't write a detailed scientific paper, but I can always clean up my desk, for example, or I can read that book I always wanted to read but never had the time for."

"I used to have many more sleepless nights than I have now and in some ways used to look forward to them," he adds. "I've been a little distressed that I just don't get that time anymore. I don't get as much reading done as I once did."

Swedish film director Ingmar Bergman uses the same tactic. He told one *New York Times* interviewer: "For the past fourteen years I can barely manage four hours of sleep a night. I've succeeded in exorcizing my insomnia thanks to books and music. I'd imagine that Tolstoy and Mozart, among others, have literally saved my life." Bergman was able to repay his debt to Mozart at least by making a film of the master's opera *The Magic Flute.*

Being a night person by choice or by insomnia does not mean you've joined an army of ghouls and zombies wandering the earth when most decent, god-fearing folk are home, fast asleep. As much as some people would like to think so, there is no "type" of night person who prefers life after sundown. On the one extreme you can have someone like Gothic horror author H. P. Lovecraft, probably most famous for his eerie-weird classic, "The Strange Case of Charles Dexter Ward." From his childhood, Lovecraft was a night person. According to his biographer, L. Sprague De Camp, there were different theories about why he was this way. One claimed Lovecraft believed the night stirred imagination and freed him from distractions. Another was that Lovecraft believed his mother's claim that he was too hideous to go out in the daytime. What was more likely, says De Camp, was that Lovecraft just happened to be a night person by natural inclination. He did all his work and all his socializing at night and, on the rare occasions when he had to work in the day, he pulled down all shades and worked by lamplight.

At the other extreme, you have Elvis Presley. He routinely woke at noon and never went to bed until 4:00 A.M. He followed his night body clock no matter where he was. For example, on one occasion when he had to spend some time in a hospital, he had the windows in his room covered with aluminum foil so he could sleep during the day.

In addition to those who naturally prefer night, there is another kind of night person, the one who is in it for the money. This is the much-maligned night-shift worker, who, according to all the experts, is doomed to a miserable working and social life. The problem with so many of the people who study night people is that they are usually speaking from a biased viewpoint. For example, one University of Michigan sociologist who spent three years working on a night shift herself described night people as antisocial loners who seldom dated and who avoided parties, preferring to cling to their neurotic way of life. Typically, she reported, night people withdraw from the world of their day friends and instead build up a society of new "night" friends. Among the strange behavior she observed among night people was that they were "honest and open" with each other; "they had to interact and receive human warmth and definition from each other"; and "herculean efforts were made to keep conflicts smoothed over and outcasts usually left night work."

Another problem with scientific studies about night workers is that they keep carefully tabulated number counts of how many people are working nights and make long shopping lists of the effects of the kinds of ailments that plague the night worker—digestive problems, leg and foot cramps, colds, chest pains, menstrual problems, shakiness, problems with booze and pills, fatigue—but, if you take a look at the details of the articles, you find that they often lump shift workers in with night workers. This is definitely an apples and oranges mix, for the simple reason that night workers follow a steady, routine part of the twenty-four-hour day, while shift workers have their work time and body time changed every month or so, causing chaos with their internal clocks.

"It doesn't make that much difference to our bodies how we put the twenty-four-hour cycle together," says one sleep researcher, "as long as there is a consistency to it. What is hell is all that switching." Because of the confusion between shift work and night work, many people mistakenly pin the blame for their problems on being up at night and not the fact that they've been abusing their body rhythms by hopping around the clock.

This is not to say that there are no problems that come with working nights. A marriage with a day-shift wife and night-shift husband usually suffers from the kind of seesaw life-style that goes with it. The only solution is for both to go on the same time schedule. And when there is a showdown about who is going to change whose shift or schedule, more often than not the night person loses out.

A night person with a family is probably the one who suffers most of all, trying to juggle, usually unsuccessfully, his or her night work schedule during the week with a day schedule on weekends so he or she can see spouse and children.

In spite of these drawbacks, night work does have some advantages, as many businesses now know. According to the U.S. Department of Labor, the number of people working on evening and night shifts, so-called nonstandard work shifts, is now close to 10 million. One reason is, with the energy crisis and the higher utility bills it has spawned, many businesses have now shifted some of their operations to off-peak hours to take advantage of lower nighttime rates. Other businesses simply keep their operations going twenty-four hours per day as part of their zeal to make more money.

Night-shift workers can benefit from this around-the-clock frenzy by the higher salaries paid on that shift. They can also enjoy the fringe benefits of having the day to do with as they wish, whether it's running errands or just relaxing in the sun. And, for all the problems of night work, they are free from the typical headaches of the day worker: rush-hour traffic to and from work, frantic lunch-hour scrambles for places to eat, and shopping trips shoehorned into a tight day-time schedule.

For some night people there is also that intangible which won't show up on any study or report on living and working at night: the fact that some of them like it. For example, there's Carol, a twenty-seven-year-old "ex-guidance counsellor" who went back to school to become a computer programer so she could make more money. As a novice programer she was first put on the night shift. She found she liked it so much that she stayed there and advanced quickly in her job, since the competition was not as stiff for supervisory night work. "At first I did it for the money," she says, "but after a while I found it suited me. I found I was a nocturnal person."

What about the dreary existence of the night owl? "I have lots of friends who are night people. I meet them on my job or at the after-hours disco where I go to unwind." And as for insomnia? "It hasn't bothered me that much. I simply don't go to bed if I'm not tired," she says. "My main problem is overcoming the worry about not getting enough sleep. If you can get your mind off that, you've won half the battle."

Her personal fail-safe solution to the problem is also a highly orig-inal one. "I create stories out of the thoughts that come into my head," she explains. "It began one night when I couldn't sleep because someone very close to me had died. All these thoughts started creeping into my head, so I decided to write them down in the form of a story about him. The result, I thought, was very poetic, and after I finished I fell peacefully asleep."

"The whole thing started by accident," she explained. "I had a habit of keeping pen and paper by my bed to write down my dreams because I wanted to tell them to my analyst. Even after I quit analysis, I kept the habit."

"When I do this," she added, "I can't go to sleep until every last word is perfect in my mind. I'm very particular about every word; the whole process of writing is like a lullaby to me."

It's probably safe to say that, while night people are not loners, they are a special breed of independent people who thrive on pursuing the unusual, the esoteric, helping us in some instances to broaden our knowledge of ourselves (as in sleep research) and our universe. One good example of the independent types is Charles Kowal, an astronomer who's famous in his field for several reasons. Before he reached his mid-thirties he had already discovered two new moons around the planet Jupiter, the first new moons of any kind discovered in the past quarter-century; he logged the second highest number of sightings of exploding stars, called supernovas, in astronomical history; he found four lost comets; and most recently he spotted four miniplanet-type asteroids, one of which now bears his name. In a time in history when the space around the earth is cluttered with all kinds of observatory satellites, and when sophisticated radio telescopes are in use, Kowal made his discoveries in the simple, old-fashioned way, by looking through the eyepiece of one of the Hale Observatory telescopes in California. He is also one of the few professional astronomers with only a bachelor's degree, which is extremely rare in a field where a Ph.D. is standard academic equipment.

For seven nights every month he works ten and a half hours at a stretch, peering through the telescope at stars, planets, and asteroids, always looking for a new surprise in space. It's often grueling, painstaking work, involving just him, the stars, and the night. And it suits him fine. "In my kind of job, you don't become famous or rich," he told one reporter, "but I'm doing exactly what I want to do with my life. That makes me one of the happiest men on earth."

Night people are not all the dreary, miserable drones we might like to think they are. Many of them are out there having a good time, enjoying life, and, many times, keeping things working smoothly as well. After all, night people are the ones who patrol your city streets after dark; who are ready to take care of you in hospital emergency rooms all over the country; who make sure you're getting your share of heat, power, and water around the clock; who pick up your garbage; who make your morning paper possible; and who entertain you (what would 16 million people do if Johnny Carson decided to go on a day shift?).

To help you appreciate them and their world, heed this little bit of advice: "Listen to them—the children of the night. What music they make!" And this, from someone who should know—Count Dracula.

Appendix

SLEEP CLINICS

If you feel your insomnia is serious enough to need professional attention, consult your doctor first. If one of your doctor's remedies help, then it may be time to call in the heavy artillery. Sleep clinics are fairly new on the medical scene, so you may have trouble finding one near you, or your doctor may not even be aware that such a thing exists. To give you some assistance, here's a state-by-state listing of some places that might be able to tackle your sleep problem. Policies vary from one clinic to another regarding whether or not you have to be referred for treatment by your doctor. You might want to write first for information about what standard procedure is.

ALABAMA
UAB Sleep Clinic
University of Alabama Medical Center
University Station
Birmingham, Alabama 35294
ATTN: Vernon Pegrem, M.D.

ARKANSAS
Sleep Disorders Clinic
c/o Department of Neurosurgery
University of Arkansas for Medical Sciences
Little Rock, Arkansas 72201
ATTN: Herman Flanigan, M.D.

CALIFORNIA
Sleep Disorders Unit
University of California School of Medicine
San Francisco, California 94101
ATTN: Jean-Paul Spire, M.D.

Sleep Disorders Center
Stanford University Medical Center
Stanford, California 94305
ATTN: William C. Dement, M.D.

Department of Medicine
University of California Irvine Medical Center
101 City Drive South
Orange, California 92688
ATTN: Jon F. Sassin, M.D.

Southern California Center for Sleep Disorders
Suite 1402
Santa Monica, California 90404
ATTN: John Beck, M.D.

Sleep Disorders Clinic
Department of Psychiatry
Veterans Administration Hospital
3350 La Jolla Village Drive
San Diego, California 92161
ATTN: Daniel Kripke, M.D.

FLORIDA
Mt. Sinai Medical Center

4300 Alton Beach
Miami Beach, Florida 33140
ATTN: Marvin Sachner, M.D.

LOUISIANA
Department of Psychiatry and Neurology
Tulane Medical School
1430 Tulane Ave.
New Orleans, Louisiana 70112
ATTN: John W. Goethe, M.D.

MARYLAND
Department of Psychiatry
Baltimore City Hospital
Baltimore, Maryland 21224
ATTN: Richard P. Allen, M.D.

MASSACHUSETTS
Department of Neurology
University of Massachusetts
55 Lake Avenue
Worcester, Massachusetts 01605
ATTN: Sheldon Kapen, M.D.

Boston State Hospital
591 Morton Street
Boston, Massachusetts 02124
ATTN: Ernest Hartmann, M.D.

Sleep Clinic
Peter Bent Brigham Hospital and New Center of Psychotherapies
721 Huntington Avenue
Boston, Massachusetts 02115
ATTN: Quentin Regestein, M.D.

NEW HAMPSHIRE
Dartmouth Sleep Clinic

Dartmouth Medical School
Hanover, New Hampshire 03755
ATTN: Peter Hauri, Ph.D.

NEW JERSEY
Sleep/Wakefulness Clinic
College of Medicine and Dentistry
100 Bergen Street
Newark, New Jersey 07102
ATTN: James Minard, Ph.D.

NEW YORK
Department of Psychiatry
Albany Medical College
Albany, New York 12208
ATTN: Vincenzo Castaldo, M.D.

Sleep-Wake Disorders Unit
Department of Neurology
Montefiore Hospital and Medical Center
111 East 210th Street
Bronx, New York 10467
ATTN: Elliot D. Weitzman, M.D.

OHIO
Sleep Disorders Evaluation Center
Ohio State University College of Medicine
473 West 12th Avenue
Columbus, Ohio 43210
ATTN: Helmut Schmidt, M.D.

University of Cincinnati Sleep Disorders Center
Veterans Administration Hospital
Sleep Lab 116-Al
3200 Vine Street
Cincinnati, Ohio 45220
ATTN: Milton Kramer, M.D.

or

University of Cincinnati Sleep Disorders Center
Christian R. Holmes Hospital
Eden and Bethesda Avenue
Cincinnati, Ohio 45219
ATTN: Frank Zorick, M.D.

OKLAHOMA
Sleep Physiology Laboratory
Veterans Administration Hospital (183A)
921 NE 13th Street
Oklahoma City, Oklahoma 73104
ATTN: William C. Orr, Ph.D.

PENNSYLVANIA
Sleep Evaluation Center
Western Psychiatric Institute and Clinic
3811 O'Hara Street
Pittsburgh, Pennsylvania 15261
ATTN: David J. Kupfer, M.D.

Sleep Research and Treatment Center
Pennsylvania State University
Milton S. Hershey Medical Center
Hershey, Pennsylvania 17033
ATTN: Anthony Kales, M.D.

TENNESSEE
Sleep Disorders Center
Baptist Memorial Hospital
899 Madison Avenue
Memphis, Tennessee 38146
ATTN: Helio Lemmi, M.D.

TEXAS
Sleep Disorders Center
Baylor College of Medicine
Houston, Texas 77025
ATTN: Ismet Karacan, M.D.

VIRGINIA
Sleep and Dream Laboratory
University of Virginia Medical Center
Charlottesville, Virginia 22901
ATTN: Robert Van de Castle, M.D.

CANADA
Sleep Disorders Center
Hospital du Sacre-Coeur
5400 Ouest, Boulevard Gouin
Montreal, Quebec
H4J 1C5, Canada
ATTN: Jacques Montplaisir, M.D.

Ottawa General Hospital
43 Bruyere
Ottawa, Ontario
K1N 5C8, Canada
ATTN: Roger J. Broughton, M.D.

Department of Clinical Neurophysiology
Clarke Institute of Psychiatry
Toronto, Canada
ATTN: Harvey Moldofsky, M.D.

BY PRESCRIPTION ONLY

This does not pretend to be a total listing of all possible sleeping pills. At last count there were over seventy drugs that qualified as hypnotics. A complete list would be much longer but probably not all that valuable, unless you plan to open your own drug store. What you'll find here are the most commonly prescribed drugs, listed by their main drug grouping, their generic names, brand names, and, to give you an idea of how long some of these have been around, the year they were introduced into medical practice. You'll notice that all the barbiturates can do double duty as either a sedative or barbiturate, depending on the dose in which they are given. In low dosages, they will relax you. In high dosages, they will make you unconscious.

DRUG GROUP	GENERIC NAME	BRAND NAMES	YEAR INTRODUCED
I. Barbiturates			
	Amobarbital (sedative/hypnotic)	Amytol Sodium Tuinal (a combination drug; mixed with secobarbital)	1925
	Butabarbital (sedative/hypnotic)	Bubartal Butisol Sodium	1939
	Pentobarbital (sedative/hypnotic)	Carbrital Nembutal Night-Caps	1930
	Phenobarbital (sedative/hypnotic)	Luminal Stental	1912
	Secobarbital (sedative/hypnotic)	Seconal Tuinal (with amobarbital)	1936
II. Nonbarbiturates			
	Chloral hydrate	Dormal Noctec Somnos	1860
	Ethchlorvynol	Placidyl	1956
	Glutethimide	Doriden Dorimide	1954
	Methaqualone	Parest Quaalude Sopor Somnafac	1965
	Methyprylon	Noludar	1955
III. Benzodiazepines			
	Flurazepam	Dalmane	1970

Index